Contemplating the Role of an Intensive Care Doctor

Diane Dennis • Peter Vernon van Heerden
Michael Ruppe

Editors

Contemplating the Role of an Intensive Care Doctor

A Fieldwork Guide to Intensive
Care Medicine

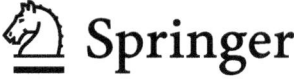 Springer

Editors
Diane Dennis
Departments of Intensive Care and
Physiotherapy
Sir Charles Gairdner Osborne Park
Healthcare Group
Perth, WA, Australia

Peter Vernon van Heerden
Department of Anesthesiology
Critical Care and Pain Medicine
Hadassah University Medical Center
Jerusalem, Israel

Michael Ruppe
University of Louisville Department
of Pediatrics, Division of Critical Care,
and Norton Children's Medical Group
Louisville, KY, USA

ISBN 978-3-031-92765-2   ISBN 978-3-031-92766-9   (eBook)
https://doi.org/10.1007/978-3-031-92766-9

This Springer imprint is published by the registered company Springer Nature Switzerland AG
The registered company address is: Gewerbestrasse 11, 6330 Cham, Switzerland

If disposing of this product, please recycle the paper.

Preface

There is no one set of answers suitable for everyone (PV van Heerden, "Stories from ICU Doctors", 2023)

Each of us has a unique set of personal characteristics that define our capability in any circumstance. The ancient Greek maxim "know thyself" reflects the notion of exploring and analyzing our authentic selves to identify both our aspirations and limitations. Self-reflection is perhaps key to unlocking our potential—searching and investigating our individual thoughts, feelings, and responses in any given scenario. This book aims to provide fodder for the deliberate self-reflection of doctors working or intending to work within the intensive care environment to elicit preparatory insight, meaning, growth, and self-awareness. Sometimes this self-reflection will be best done in isolation; sometimes it will work best in consultation with mentors.

In our first book, *Stories from ICU Doctors* [1], we explored the reflections of more than 45 experienced intensivists relating to the stressors involved in working in the intensive care environment. The book provided a broad overview of contemporary issues and, to some extent, sought to normalize the experiences, responses, and coping strategies commonly employed.

In this follow-up book, the everyday real-time experiences and concerns of those intensivists have been distilled down to more than 100 quotations across four parts. In Part I, we place this book in the context of a pragmatic "fieldwork guide" for doctors beginning their career within the critical care environment. We explain how readers might use the book as trainees in the field (Chap. 1); within the constructs of meta-communication and meta-cognition (Chap. 2), or in a mentoring relationship (Chap. 3); and we consider ethics (Chap. 4) and the psychology of readers related to the themes that will be subsequently examined (Chap. 5).

In Part II, we dive into the metaphorical waters of ICU and begin to swim. In these five chapters, the authors constructed a series of dot-point statements around quotations extracted from our original dataset to provoke the thoughtful contemplation of the reader. We explore the personality traits and role of the intensive care doctor (Chaps. 6 and 7), and the environment both within and external to the intensive care unit (Chaps. 8, 9, and 10). The authors in Part III used the same approach over 4 chapters to have readers reflect on communication scenarios in intensive care medicine. How do doctors sing from the same songbook (Chap. 11); stay in harmony with others (Chap. 12); perform to different audiences (Chap. 13); and when required, lead the choir (Chap. 14)?

Part IV offers a guide to the maintenance of the psychological safety of the reader during their reflections and beyond into the real world of clinical practice, using the allegorical context of aerial acrobatics. We consider mastery—reflecting on those learning to climb the ropes (Chap. 15); those dealing with unexpected changes in routine (Chap. 16); and the safety nets that are needed throughout the whole performance of working as a leader in the intensive care environment (Chap. 17). In closing we set the scene to bounce safely off the net, forward (Chap. 18).

The current editorial group would like to extend their grateful thanks to our colleagues who contributed to our first book *Stories from ICU Doctors* [1], especially our co-editors on the project—Aaron Calhoun, Rahul Khanna, and Cameron Knott. We and our authors also gratefully acknowledge the magnanimous contribution of research study participants who shared their reflections about their work in the intensive care specialty with honesty and candor. Their unidentified verbatim quotations have been used throughout the text to facilitate the reader's consideration. This work was supported by the Charlies Foundation for Research, the Raine Medical Research Foundation, and the Sir Charles Gairdner Osborne Park Healthcare Group within the North Metropolitan Health Service, in Perth, Western Australia.

Perth, WA, Australia   Diane Dennis
Jerusalem, Israel   Peter Vernon van Heerden
Louisville, KY, USA   Michael Ruppe
February 2025

Reference

1. Dennis, D., Calhoun, A., Knott, C., Khanna, R., and van Heerden, P.V. (Eds.). "Stories from ICU doctors: navigating and conquering adversity" (2023).

Contents

About the Editors and Contributors

About the Editors

Diane Dennis has been employed as a researcher in the ICU setting since 2008, with an interest in simulation and human factors in the safe delivery of healthcare services. She has been exploring the well-being of medical staff in the specialty since 2018. With a background in clinical training as a physiotherapist, she taught as Co-lead of Simulation and Senior Lecturer at Curtin University; worked as an Allied Health and Research Coordinator; and is currently the Head of the Physiotherapy Department at Sir Charles Gairdner Osborne Park Healthcare Group in Perth, Western Australia. She has recently been consulting for the College of Intensive Care Medicine of Australia and New Zealand Rural Trainee mentoring programme.

Peter Vernon van Heerden qualified as an anaesthetist and intensive care specialist and has practiced in South Africa, the United Kingdom, Australia and Israel. He is the Director of the Department of General Intensive Care, Faculty of Medicine, Hadassah Hospital and Hebrew University of Jerusalem, Israel, and a full professor of anaesthesiology and critical care at the Hebrew University of Jerusalem.

Michael Ruppe is a Professor in the Department of Pediatrics at the University of Louisville School of Medicine and an attending physician in Pediatric Cardiac Critical Care at Norton Children's Hospital, Louisville, Kentucky, USA. His research interests include end-of-life decision-making, medical ethics, intubation safety and pediatric cardiac critical care. He serves as medical director of the pediatric critical care point-of-care ultrasound program and his clinical passions include quality improvement in the care of patients with congenital heart disease, and international health.

About the Contributors

Qalab Abbas is an Associate Professor and pediatric intensivist at the Aga Khan University & Hospital, Karachi. His research focuses on respiratory care in low-resource settings, quality improvement and use of predictive analytics in pediatric critical care. Dr Abbas is dedicated to enhancing Pediatric Intensive Care Unit (PICU) capacity building and advancing care for critically ill children in his own country and low-resource settings through innovative research and clinical excellence.

Aaron Calhoun is a tenured Professor in the Department of Pediatrics, Division of Pediatric Critical Care at the University of Louisville, and is an attending physician in the Just for Kids Critical Care Center at Norton Children's Hospital. He received his MD from Johns Hopkins University School of Medicine in 2001, completed general pediatrics residency at Children's Memorial Hospital/Northwestern University Feinberg School of Medicine in 2004 and completed pediatric critical care fellowship at Children's Hospital of Boston/Harvard School of Medicine in 2007. Dr Calhoun is the Division Chief of Pediatric Critical Care and has numerous publications in the field of simulation and medical education.

Christopher Danbury trained in general internal medicine, microbiology, virology and anaesthesia before switching to intensive care medicine. Appointed a consultant in 2002, his practice is in General and Neurological Intensive Care Medicine. His current clinical base is at the University Hospital Southampton, the United Kingdom. He has academic roles at the University of Southampton, Kings College London and the University of Reading. His research interests are in complex decision-making related to serious medical treatment and the interface between law and medicine. He has held national leadership roles and sat on a number of national guideline development groups.

Eric Eisenberg is Professor of Communication and Senior Vice President of University Community Partnerships at the University of South Florida. Eisenberg graduated Phi Beta Kappa from Rutgers University and received his doctorate in Organizational Communication from Michigan State University. Dr Eisenberg is the author of over 50 articles, chapters and books on organizational and health communication with his most recent work focused on handoffs and the role of communication in promoting patient safety. Dr Eisenberg is an internationally recognized consultant specializing in the strategic use of communication to shape organizational culture and promote positive organizational change.

Jamie Furlong-Dillard is an Associate Professor in the Department of Pediatrics, Division of Pediatric Critical Care at the University of Louisville. She completed medical school at the Virginia College of Osteopathic Medicine and completed pediatric residency at the University of Arkansas School of Medicine and pediatric critical care fellowship at the University of Utah. She is the ECMO medical director and research medical director and works as a pediatric cardiac critical care intensivist with a research focus on ECMO and cardiac nutrition.

Denise Goodman trained in pediatrics at Cincinnati Children's Hospital Medical Center and pediatric critical care at Children's Hospital of Pittsburgh. Prior to this, she had undertaken a BS (Physics) at Niagara University and her MD at the State University of NY at Buffalo (now Jacobs School of Medicine at University at Buffalo). She has also earned a MS Epidemiology at Harvard T.H. Chan School of Public Health. She spent the academic year 2012–2013 as the Morris Fishbein Fellow in Medical Editing at JAMA. Her interests include delivery of care, outcomes, care of children with medical complexity and medical editing. She considers it a privilege to accompany children and their families through some of the most difficult experiences in their lives and to share both their joys and challenges.

Bertrand Guidet is the past director of the Medical Intensive Care at the Hôpital Saint Antoine in Paris, France. In 1987, he joined the Medical Intensive Care Board. In 1993, he gained the necessary qualifications to perform research direction. He has been a university medical professor since 1997. Professor Guidet is a member of the research unit INSERM U1136 at the National Institute for Health and Medical Research (INSERM), which is a French public organization entirely dedicated to biological, medical and public health research. He is the past President (2008–2010) of the French Society for Intensive Care. He is a member of the Health Research and Services outcome section of the European Society of Intensive Care Medicine (ESICM). He is involved with the French ministry of health on ICU organization at the national level. Professor Guidet has written 481 articles published in national and international journals. He was the PI of several national and international studies. He is member of the National Medical Academia.

Zena Leah Harris currently serves as Professor and Chair of the Department of Pediatrics for the Dell Medical School at the University of Texas at Austin, Director of the Dell Pediatric Research Institute and Physician-in-Chief at Dell Children's Medical Center. She is a proud practicing Pediatric Critical Care Medicine physician, lifelong learner and multidisciplinary supporter.

Laura Hawryluck is a Professor of Critical Care Medicine in the Inter-Departmental Critical Care Medicine Program (IDDCM) the University of Toronto, Canada. She was Physician Lead of Critical Care Rapid Response Team at Toronto Western Hospital and was Corporate Chair of the Acute Resuscitation Committee at University Health Network, Toronto, for over a decade. She is a past President of the Medico-Legal Society of Toronto (MLST). Her international work aims to develop and promote education and training in critical care medicine, end-of-life decision-making and care, medico-legal issues, policy and quality improvement initiatives. She was awarded the Queen's Golden Jubilee Medal for contributions to Canada for improving end-of-life care for Canadians, the MLST award for contributions to law and medicine and the IDDCM's Humanitarian award. She has authored and co-edited *The Law of Acute Care Medicine* (Thomson Reuters), four books of poetry *An ICU Doctor's Reflections*, *Words that Matter* and *ICU Pandemic Diary* , *Our Stories* (Olympia Publishers, UK) and co-edited the book *Pandemic Voices: Untold Stories from the Frontlines* (University of Toronto Press, Canada).

Andrew Holt has worked in Critical Care for over 40 years. He graduated with MBBS (1980 Melbourne) and commenced Anaesthesia training within the Austin programme. He rapidly fell in love with pathophysiology and re-directed his training to ICU, principally at Flinders Medical Centre, Adelaide. He completed both his Anaesthetic (ANZCA 1990) and ICU (CICM 1988) training. Dr Holt subsequently completed dual certification in pediatric ICU at the Royal Children's Hospital, Melbourne. He returned to Flinders Medical Centre and was instrumental in setting up the Cardiac Surgical and Liver Transplant programmes at Flinders Medical Centre. Dr Holt has been Director of the South Australian Home Parenteral Nutrition Unit for over 30 year and has more than 80 peer-reviewed publications. Outside work, Dr Holt loves wilderness, and he is acknowledged as the worst Kayaker to have successfully completed a Bass Strait crossing.

Carl Horsley is a dual trained intensivist currently working in the Critical Care Complex of Middlemore Hospital, Auckland, New Zealand. He is also the Clinical Lead for System Safety at Te Tāhū Hauora (Health Quality and Safety Commission) and is leading work to introduce modern safety science approaches into healthcare in Aotearoa, New Zealand; Dr Horsley recently completed his MSc in Human Factors and System Safety at Lund University, Sweden, with a focus on the sociology of safety.

Melanie Jansen is a Pediatric Intensive Care Specialist and Clinical Ethicist. Her clinical interests are in cardiac intensive care and ECMO, retrieval and the management of severe trauma. She is also interested in staff well-being, teamwork and relational skills, and real-time ethics at the bedside, including the ethics of end-of-life care and organ donation. She has a Master of Arts in Philosophy and completed a Churchill Fellowship in clinical ethics and medical humanities in 2017. She is a PhD candidate at the University of Queensland, developing a pedagogy for complex decision-making skills in critical care. Melanie currently works in PICU at the Queensland Children's Hospital and is the Clinical Ethicist for Gold Coast Hospital and Health Service.

Kylie Julian is an intensivist at the Department of Critical Care Medicine, Auckland. She is interested in the experience of all those who intersect with intensive care—clinicians, patients and their families. She is the medical lead for teams that follow up patients who survive critical illness in her unit, and the families of those who do not. She set up and coordinates the Auckland Regional Intensive Care Mentoring Programme, which links intensive care trainees with intensivist mentors. Along with her colleagues Dr Laura Tincknell and Dr Ravi Mistry, she co-convenes the Intensive Care Part 3 Course. This course equips senior intensive care trainees with skills and knowledge to thrive in the transition from trainee to specialist.

Rakesh Khanna works as a full-time Consultant Psychiatrist at Northpark Hospital in Victoria. He has previously worked in several public and private practice settings. He was the Director of Clinical Services at the Austin and Repatriation Medical Centre from June 1998 to February 2002 and at the Bendigo and Regional Mental Health Services, Bendigo, from April 1996 to June 1998. He was a Lecturer and Honorary Senior Fellow at Melbourne University. 2001 to 2011 and Assistant and Associate Professor of Psychiatry from March 1987 to February 1995 at the Central Institute of Psychiatry, Kanke, Ranchi, India. He has extensive experience in clinical, teaching and research and has published more than 40 articles in various peer-reviewed journals.

Roxanne Kirsch joined the Hospital for Sick Children, Toronto, in 2016. She is co-appointed to the Department of Critical Care Medicine, Division of Cardiac Critical Care and the Department of Bioethics. In June 2023, Dr Kirsch was appointed Chief for the Division of Cardiac Critical Care, having served as Interim Chief since January 2022. In addition, she is Associate Chief of the Department of Perioperative Services for Equity, Diversity, Inclusiveness, Wellness and Faculty Development. She has completed a Master's degree in Biomedical Ethics at the University of Pennsylvania. Dr Kirsch's academic work focuses on the ethical and social challenges of stopping advanced technologic therapies, end-of-life care, introduction of innovative therapies and resource allocation and prioritization. Additionally, she works to educate clinicians and enhance their facility with ethical issues intendant to pediatric critical care and cardiology to improve patient care delivery.

Kelly Lyons is a pediatric intensive care and pediatric palliative care attending physician at the Just for Kids Critical Care Center and Pediatric Support Team at Norton Children's Hospital, University of Louisville School of Medicine. She received her medical degree from the Lake Erie College of Osteopathic Medicine in 2014; completed an Internal Medicine and Pediatrics residency at the University of Buffalo School of Medicine in 2018, where she was Chief Resident from 2017–2018; and completed pediatric critical care fellowship at University of Louisville in 2021. Dr Lyons is an Assistant Professor at the University of Louisville School of Medicine and has research interests in palliative care medicine, medical education and communication research.

Mary Pinder is an Intensive Care Specialist and Director of Clinical Training based at Sir Charles Gairdner Hospital in Perth, Western Australia. She trained in intensive care in the UK and South Africa as well as Australia. She is on the Board of the College of Intensive Care Medicine and roles with CICM have included Chair of the Second Part Exam Committee, Chair of the Assessments Committee and College President.

Kenneth Remy is an Associate Professor in the Divisions of Pulmonary Critical Care Medicine and Pediatric Critical Care Medicine at University Hospitals of Cleveland/Rainbow Babies and Children's Hospital in Cleveland, Ohio, USA. He is Director of the Division of Pulmonary Critical Care Medicine Basic Science and Translational Critical Care Research and Co-director for Clinical, Basic Science, and Translational Critical Care Research in the Division of Pediatric Critical Care Medicine. His expertise lies in adult and pediatric sepsis, COVID disease and global health. He has been featured on a number of news programmes including CNN, BBC News and Reuters on his experiences during this pandemic and has been speaking on the immunologic consequences of disease, pediatric multisystem inflammatory syndrome (MIS-C), public health measures and schools and potential therapies for SARS-CoV-2 infection.

Kerry Strayer teaches courses in teamwork, leadership and organizational communication. She has worked as a consultant on board leadership and organizational change in both non-profit and for-profit organizations. Her most recent scholarship focuses on how medical schools teach cultural competency skills.

Eileen Tay is a Consultant Psychiatrist, Clinical Senior Lecturer and Clinical Subdean (MD2 year) in Perth, Australia. She is interested in developing further supervision skills for medical practitioners and is currently undertaking additional training in this field of work, as supervision is an increasingly recognised discipline in the helping professions. She has been involved in doctors' health for over 20 years as part of an advisory and treating clinician network. She is also developing comparative Psychotherapy education modules for psychiatry trainees.

Luke Torre is an Australian trained ICU specialist and Anaesthetist who works in Perth, Western Australia. He has an extensive involvement in teaching and clinical work during his 25-year medical career (ongoing). Luke is married with five school-aged children and is a strong believer in Catholic moral teaching, namely, where your treasure is there your heart will be also.

Adam van Heerden Trained as an Educational and Developmental Psychologist, Adam supports clients across the lifespan. He runs his private practice, Inner Spark Psychology, in Naarm/Melbourne, Australia, and serves as a bereavement counsellor in community palliative care, where he approaches his work with humility and respect for the profound experiences of clients and their families.

Part I
User's Guide to This Book

Foreword: How to Use a Crystal Ball

Diane Dennis

> With high hope for the future, no prediction is ventured. (Abraham Lincoln)

Many people view fortune tellers purely as entertainers who use tricks and illusions without any true gift of prophecy. Despite this, to some extent, we likely all reflect on what the future has in store for us. We gaze forward with excitement and sometimes nervous anticipation about what is around the corner, and we can in this sense, all buff our shiny crystal ball to prepare as best we can for what lies ahead! But where can we each find our own metaphorical crystal ball? We offer this book as a sphere on which the reader may focus their thoughts to concentrate on the things relevant to a future working within the intensive care specialty. Thoughtful contemplation will allow the reader to polish, place and consider their ball without harming themselves. The following five introductory chapters provide a user's guide as to how the book can help to do this.

In Chap. 1, we begin polishing our crystal ball by talking about where an intensive care unit sits within a tertiary hospital in terms of its role and relationship with other areas; what the environment is like; and what an intensivist does. We also discuss in broad terms what the training pathway looks like for doctors entering the field. In the next chapter, we talk about where to place the ball. An individual needs to be able to step away and consider from where they gaze, thinking about thinking. They need to create an awareness of their own understanding and performance by looking deep within themselves.

Although we often need to ponder the future alone, it is sometimes more helpful to share what you see coming with others. In Chap. 3, we consider who else is sitting at the table crystal gazing with you. This is especially important when the crystal ball appears clouded—people who have travelled down the road before you may know the way and be able to offer a clear route through the haze with their perspective and sage advice. In Chap. 4, we consider the ethics of working in the intensive care environment—both knowing and then doing what is right. The dangers of too much ball-gazing are discussed in Chap. 5. We suggest you read this carefully to prepare yourself to use the book appropriately. Self-reflection is important, but overthinking can be harmful.

While there is no doubt that many people claim to see visions in crystal balls, we have used them here as an analogy to describe a practice of deep reflection, alone or with others, that will enable one to deliberate and predict the success of a future career path within the ICU specialty.

Chapter 1
So, You Want to Be an ICU Doctor? How This Book Might Be Useful for an ICU Trainee

Roxanne Kirsch (iD) **and Jamie Furlong-Dillard**

> *Learn from many but copy none.*
> —*Mark Sanborn*

The "intensive care unit" (ICU) is a cornerstone of the modern tertiary hospital. The sickest of patients will come through the ICU, often on a long journey of care for congenital and acquired diseases that will be life-long. For some diseases, the intensiveness of therapy in infancy and early childhood is particularly intense, such as that for congenital heart disease or congenital diaphragmatic hernia. The patients may come to the ICU from the emergency department, from any ward in the hospital, or from outside hospitals seeking support in escalating care for the very sickest. As the centre of stabilization and rescue for all patients, the ICU team must be able to rapidly assess and coordinate care in an unpredictable daily flow, as there may be multiple patients in need of rescue or stretches of minimal activity. Patients could have planned recoveries from surgical services or after certain medical treatments, post-transplant, or unplanned emergent admissions such as trauma, ingestions, or acute infection. Often the ICU may be a monitoring environment in preparation for potential acute decompensations or deteriorations [1]. Generally, ICU services are triaged so that the sickest patients are within the physical ICU. There are also extensions of the ICU environment that exist in consulting services where doctors and nurses with intensive care skills review and consult on patients who are in non-ICU environments to support and monitor for the need to escalate to the ICU or to

R. Kirsch (✉)
Department of Critical Care Medicine, Hospital for Sick Children, Toronto, ON, Canada

The Department of Bioethics, The Hospital for Sick Children, Toronto, Canada
e-mail: roxanne.kirsch@sickkids.ca

J. Furlong-Dillard
University of Louisville Department of Pediatrics and Norton Children's Medical Group, Louisville, KY, USA
e-mail: jamie.furlong-dillard@louisville.edu

3

provide interventions to prevent worsening of illness and requirement for ICU. Since the support in a tertiary hospital is also that of a referral centre, ICU is responsible for bringing the sickest patients from outside hospitals to the site of intensive care. This then means that mini teams are sent out via multiple transport methods to initiate stabilization and bring patients to ICU in a timely fashion for the most advanced care and rescue.

The term "intensive care unit" invokes images of very ill patients surrounded by the latest in biomedical equipment, monitoring devices, sterile settings and code carts. There are a variety of ICU settings and types of critical care units, including medical and surgical ICUs, as well as highly specialized units such as cardiovascular, transplant, neurological and burn units. Despite the variation in setting, bed space and unit design, the ICU environment is a high-stakes, fast-paced space that demands constant vigilance and quick decision-making from medical professionals.

The visual aspect of the ICU is dominated by the presence of medical equipment and monitors. There is a constant presence of various machines such as ventilators, intravenous pumps and physiologic monitoring screens. The sounds of the ICU are the constant humming of medical equipment, bubbling of chest tubes, chirping of telemetry or ventilator alarms, opening and closing of doors and the undulating rhythm of staff conversations. The sounds not heard are the constant internal dialogue of an ICU physician. The smell of an ICU is often characterized by the scent of antiseptics, cleaning agents and medical supplies. Patients experience touch through medical interventions and examinations that occur at any time of the day. In the ICU, patients often face life-threatening conditions that require immediate attention, no matter the time of day or day of the week. Physicians must assess constant changes in a patient's condition and make complex and quick decisions regarding their treatment. This urgency is at times heightened by the complex and unstable nature of critically sick patients. The non-stop nature of the ICU ensures that any sudden changes in a patient's condition are immediately addressed, regardless of the time of day or night. Physicians in the ICU must rely on their expertise, their team and their experiences to make crucial decisions under pressure.

Often physicians in the ICU spend most of their day communicating with others. The role of communication in the ICU is fundamental to ensuring patient safety, coordinating care, enhancing decision-making, supporting patients and families, managing expectations and facilitating continuity of care. ICU care is multidisciplinary, involving specialists from various fields who collaborate to create comprehensive treatment plans tailored to each patient's unique needs [2, 3]. Shared decision-making is critical in the ICU to achieve the best possible outcomes. Effective communication and coordination from each member of the care team also play a vital role in the care and recovery of patients. As the leader of the ICU, an intensivist holds the ultimate responsibility and is consistently navigating the influx of new information to decide the next best steps for their patient. Some days this is a flight or fight mechanism of response to an ever-changing patients' status where you operate under algorithms and instinct. Some days this is navigating multiple opinions from team members on next best steps while modelling professionalism and empathy to team members, and some days this is having difficult conversations related to what death may look like.

To become an intensive care physician, one must do additional specialized training. Training pathways may differ based on country and licensing or certification requirements. In general intensivists develop skills specific to the triage and prioritization of critical illness, the abilities to resuscitate emergently and adeptly use life-sustaining devices and procedures to reverse or alter a course of illness. They also need to learn skills to provide high-quality end-of-life care. For most, there is additional training following primary training in pediatrics or anaesthesiology most commonly, although certain specialists may first train as surgeons or subspecialty pediatrics (such as cardiology or pulmonology) prior to entering the training environment of an ICU. Some colleges have recognized intensive care (or critical care medicine) as its own subspecialty with board certification examinations, and specific training requirements and other programs do not have specific designations, but rather experiential and proven qualifications for practice. For most high-income countries, the ICU is solely a tertiary entity, and practices locate to urban, high population centres, although some smaller ICU or increased acuity units exist in more rural centres as well. The focus of most training programs, regardless of location, is procedurally and medically focused with the emotional toll, self-care and psychological impacts of being an intensivist left to self-discovery and experiential development.

Throughout this book we aim to help with the self-reflection and self-care necessary to understanding and adapting to the environment, pace and requirements of a career in intensive care. There are many aspects of adaptation that will strike differently at different phases of career and experience. Certainly, in the very early exposure to ICU medicine, some of the most strikingly difficult situations are those rescues which end in death or situations in which withdrawal of life-sustaining therapy takes place. While such scenarios never become easy, those with more experience have developed personal skills and methods along with ways of reflecting that minimize the impact and trauma of such experiences. Early in a career in intensive care, one also lacks the experience to have the perspective of the cases in which recovery both within and more often outside the ICU environment exceeds expectations. This too can be a point of both self-reflection and a time where shared perspectives from those more experienced can be helpful.

One might note, though, that increasingly intensive care professionals are realizing the benefits of psychotherapy and other cognitive or mindfulness activities to help deal with the emotional tolls, even at advanced stages of one's career [4]. Early on, trainees might show escalated behaviours of risk or poor choices outside of the work environment as a response to this exposure to intensity and life-and-death scenarios, and the profession has a higher risk of depression and suicide in the care providers, particularly physicians, than other professions. This is important to recognize so as to start a journey of reflection, resilience and healing early in one's career and to develop a culture in which the mental health of the intensivist is given key priority by the system, one's colleagues and oneself. It is hoped that this book may be one method of entering into the reflection on a "world" that is beyond explanation and as intensive in the experience for the providers as the name implies with regard to the therapies to the patients.

References

1. Marshall J, et al. What is an intensive care unit? A report of the task force of the world Federation of Societies of intensive and critical care medicine. J Crit Care. 2017;37:270–6.
2. Mackenzie CF, et al. The importance of communication in critical care. Crit Care Med. 2011;39(8):1912–20.
3. Weiss ME, Costa LL, Yakusheva OM, Costa LL. Communication and collaboration in critical care: a qualitative study. Crit Care Nurse. 2014;34(2):32–40.
4. Dodek, et al. Moral distress and other wellness measures in Canadian critical care physicians. AATS. 2021;18(8):1343–51.

Chapter 2
Thinking About Thinking: How This Book Might Be Useful Related to Communicating in ICU

Eric Eisenberg (iD) **and Kerry Strayer**

> *Whether you think you can or think you can't, you're right.*
> —*Henry Ford*

As an intensivist, you are thrust into the role of leader of a clinical team responsible for the most challenging cases in the hospital. You have earned this role because you have excellent technical skills and knowledge; however, this does not necessarily mean you have mastered the communication and leadership skills needed to excel.

Leadership and interpersonal mastery are less about what you know about communication and more about your daily practice; unfortunately, intelligence and communicative competence are only weakly correlated. Improving communicative practice must always begin with honest self-reflection. It is only when one develops a deep appreciation for how their communication is perceived by others that true improvement is possible. Mastering communication therefore requires you to embrace your role as a reflexive practitioner, someone who simultaneously does good work and monitors oneself for opportunities to improve.

The information in this book is designed to help you with this process. Our aim is to offer ways to monitor and assess your own and others' communication, provide guides to improving shared decision-making on your teams, diminish the impact of stressors and the potential for burnout, and learn the best ways to mentor new internists. We will discuss communicative practice in this chapter. The remainder of the book includes a wealth of insight and case studies from experienced intensivists to consider as you work to excel as a reflexive practitioner.

E. Eisenberg (✉)
SVP University Community Partnerships,
University of South Florida, Tampa, FL, USA
e-mail: eisenberg@usf.edu

K. Strayer
Department of Communication, Otterbein University, Westerville, OH, USA

D. Dennis et al. (eds.), *Contemplating the Role of an Intensive Care Doctor*,
https://doi.org/10.1007/978-3-031-92766-9_2

In the first section of this chapter, we define two different models of communication and show how you can use insights from each of them to improve your practice. In the section that follows, we provide a guide to looking at your own thought processes and narratives and the assumptions that underlie them. We then examine the other viewpoints, perspectives, and narratives that occur in your environment and discuss how to build shared mental models and practice heedful interaction, again culminating in improved practice and the potential for mastery.

Defining Communication

All of us communicate every single day; with our families, our colleagues, our patients, and those we pass in the hall. One communication theorist has even argued that "you cannot *not* communicate" since even when seeming to do nothing, people can take meaning from it [1]. You might pass a colleague in the hallway and be engrossed in your own thoughts and not acknowledge them; they might perceive you as rude or mad at them. You might enter a patient's room with a serious look on your face; they could presume you have bad news to deliver. You might use hospital jargon that a family member doesn't understand; they don't receive the message you intended to send. To better understand the power of communication, we will begin with two contrasting models drawn from communication theory: Communication as information transfer and communication as social construction.

Communication as Information Transfer

The lay understanding of communication is that it is a linear transmission of information that results in understanding [2]. This approach, which comes out of engineering methodologies, maintains that effective communication is the faithful and uninterrupted transmission of information that results in shared understanding [3, 4]. Put more simply, if you say, or write, something clearly and another person receives your meaning as you intended without being distracted by distortion or physical noise, you have communicated effectively.

Because poor communication is very often blamed for problems in healthcare, we will begin by applying this straightforward perspective. Consider the communication processes involved in patient or shift handover or in a myriad of other occasions for patient handoffs where information can be lost or distorted in ways that can lead to errors. If your goal is information transfer, you should be careful not to assume that because you have spoken or written something that the message has been received! All too often we send messages in ways that allow us to "check a box" that we have communicated, without any evidence that the message has landed and that our intended meaning has been grasped by the receiver. You should also consider whether the medium chosen—written or verbal orders, team meetings, and communication technology—is most likely to result in understanding. When possible, you should avoid communication passing through a long chain of individuals, much like the children's game of telephone, where details may get left out and different people's interpretations or viewpoints added.

Part of creating effective information transmission is understanding and anticipating the information needs and readiness of the receiver. What do they need to know or do? How do they prefer to receive information? Organizational theorists call this ability "heedful interrelating." It requires the message sender to become aware of what others are thinking or doing, allowing them to determine the most effective way to communicate with them.

An extension of heedful interrelating, to determine whether your communication was not only received but also understood, is a second step called "checking for grasping." Consider that:

> When preparing to throw a ball, a person will look at the intended receiver, assess the person's ability to catch it, survey the space between them, calculate the amount of force necessary to propel the ball far enough to reach the receiver. The thrower also considers any challenges (wind, trees, etc.) taking them into account, and then throws the ball, continuing to watch the ball until seeing the receiver's successful (or unsuccessful) catch. [5, p 63]

Like successfully catching the ball, communication has not actually happened until the receiver gets it—until they grasp the intended message. The true job of the sender, then, is not simply to transmit a message but also to check to see if their intended meaning has been received. Unfortunately, checking for grasping is somewhat more complicated than most people believe, because simply asking a receiver if they "got it" does not yield useful information; audiences will almost always say "yes" whether they understand or not. A better approach is to ask what a receiver plans to do with the information, which inevitably provides real evidence of grasping [5]. For your team, this may mean asking, "What are our next steps?" For a parent with a sick child, you might ask, "What part of this treatment do you think will be most difficult for your child?"

To date, most research on communication in healthcare environments has focused solely on information transmission, creating some helpful strategies. However, there is another way for clinicians to think about communication that yields different and, in some ways, deeper insights, which we will discuss next.

Communication as Social Construction

The environment and culture of the ICU—how medical teams interact, how communication with primary care doctors and with families occurs, and how patient turnover is handled—can be understood as a dynamic reality that you walk into multiple times a week. It's a given. It's how all ICUs are: complex, ever-changing, multicultural, and over-regulated. This perception allows for a certain degree of predictability.

The information transfer model described above treats communication as a process that occurs *within* an already established social context, limiting our ability to appreciate other, potentially more powerful, social dynamics. Alternately, the *social construction* approach focuses on the ways that individuals and teams use communication to create and shape the context itself. Proponents of this approach argue that communication is the primary social process through which our meaningful common world is constructed [6].

Sociologist Anthony Giddens speaks of the "duality of structure," referring both to how constraints emerge from human agency and gain power over future actions [7]. Taylor and Van Every [8] extend this idea, explaining that talk about human organizing is the continual interplay between texts (established rules and structures) and conversation (the use of these rules and structures in daily life).

What are the structures within your hospital that guide or constrain how you communicate? Is there time set aside for team meetings? Does management communicate an urgency to provide services which both conserve limited resources and yet ensure quality and safety? How do these messages and structures impact your behavior or your choices about where to spend time? Has the culture of your hospital carefully maintained the status hierarchy which exists in healthcare, making it difficult for nurses or others to speak up or challenge information from doctors? Behaviors that are repeated again and again take on a sense of inevitability, despite the fact they are human creations. The truth is that every day, and on every shift, communicative choices create or reproduce a particular culture. But because they are created by people, they can also be used to promote cultural change or establish new realities.

"Modern ICUs sit at the confluence of three major trends in healthcare: Increasing knowledge, specialization and interdependence" [9 , p 76]. No one person can keep up with all the advances and changes in medicine. This is especially true as practitioners tend to develop expertise in specific areas. Due to the complexity of the problems encountered in the ICU, team approaches are not only inevitable but advised. Teams help to combat fragmentation and complexity by engaging multiple perspectives on complex problems [10]. The social construction perspective is useful when looking at how your teams interact. How do you make sure teams are operating at their best? This is where reflecting on how your teams communicate, and the realities they perpetuate, is important.

ICU teams are interprofessional arenas, bringing in intensivists, surgeons, junior doctors, nurses, allied health professionals, and more. Each person comes with different professional training and different levels of experience. Each brings a focus or perspective based on their specialization. And, very likely, each arrives with a sense of their importance to the process and an expectation of whether their input will be taken seriously.

In doing research on what makes the best teams, Google determined that it wasn't collective IQ, socializing outside the group, or strictly following an agenda that created the best groups. It was equal distribution in conversational turn-taking, good social sensitivity, and psychological safety. The exact rules or norms a group followed were less important than the fact that a group had some rules in place.

Ideally, everyone in the group was given the opportunity to speak and was listened to respectfully. The group paid attention to how members were feeling. And critically, members perceived that the group was safe for interpersonal risk taking—that no one would be embarrassed, rejected, or punished for speaking up. Each of these elements of psychological safety requires a certain vulnerability on the part of group members and a clear flattening of the hierarchy.

Achieving this requires the team to make an effort to work together, with time set aside to reflect on situations and decisions. Individuals need to be encouraged to take initiative and to contribute their perspective. Centralized control of the group and other assumptions about how things are "supposed to work" should be minimized in exchange for taking more experimental approaches. All this processing takes time, often seen as a scarce commodity in the ICU, but the outcomes are worth it. Team members who are listened to experience less stress and burnout. Members whose opinions are given respectful consideration, even if not accepted, experience greater engagement and connection to processes.

Applying the Two Communication Models Through Reflexive Practice

Thus far in this chapter we have described two ways of thinking about communication in your clinical practice—as a means of information transmission and as an opportunity to shape local culture and shared reality. But before you can use either approach, you must first develop a deeper understanding of your current communication practices as they appear to others in the ICU setting. Some ways of doing this are described next.

Reflecting on Your Personal Narrative

According to Peter Senge [11], the individual's journey toward improvement in complex organizational systems can be expressed as the pursuit of personal mastery. Seeking personal mastery involves two related lines of reflection: continually clarifying what is most important to you and continually learning how to see current reality more clearly.

So, let's start with you. Consider your own personal narrative. What are the factors that led you to pursue a medical career? What led you to choose to be an intensivist? What is your primary focus at work? Is it to make as few errors as possible? To create a calming environment within the potential chaos of the ICU? To create the best patient experience?

You should also consider how you are "showing up" at work? Does your demeanor indicate to others that you are too busy to be interrupted? When you communicate, is it to shout orders or give commands? Even though you may ultimately be responsible for the final decision that gets made, do you sincerely ask for input? Do you take the time to listen to others who see things differently? Asking colleagues for feedback about how you appear to them as a communicator is an excellent launching point for the pursuit of greater mastery.

Reflecting on the Narratives You Share About Hospitals and Patients

Every organization is characterized by stories that are repeated over and over that express a particular view of the culture. For example: "patients can't be trusted;" "specialists are too busy to care;" or "hospital administration doesn't understand our work conditions". Over time, these stories are even passed on to new employees as part of their informal socialization. But rather than see these stories as inevitable, you can choose to selectively repeat stories that you favor and even to invent new ones. That said, introducing new narratives about patients or the hospital environment is only possible when you first take a deep dive into understanding the current narratives that are reproduced and shared without conscious thought or reflection. Like one's personal narrative, shifting the organizational narrative begins with a hard look at current reality.

Similarly, patients vary considerably in how they perceive the medical establishment and medical personnel. Are healthcare workers heroes? Is a hospital a good place which will help you or is it the end of the line? Additionally, what cultural factors are you dealing with? Are you dealing with diverse cultures? Different religious belief systems? End-of-life decisions? Patient stereotyping, while understandable, can create significant problems, and these are explored more in Chap. 9. Great communicators hold on loosely to their beliefs about people and organizations and use communication to inquire more deeply into individual differences and organizational possibilities, making deeply held assumptions and tacit beliefs more visible and therefore open for scrutiny and change.

Reflecting on the Narratives of Fellow Travelers Along the Road

While self-reflection is key to the pursuit of mastery, observing others who have done similar work and hearing their accounts of challenges, strategies, and lessons learned can be equally insightful. Closely attending to others' stories can both provide new insights and open new ways of speaking and thinking about the nature of your work. This kind of learning is at the heart of mentorship, in that it can potentially spare you from falling into common pitfalls that are well known to experienced practitioners. And while mentorship implies learning from more senior colleagues, one can also take lessons from peers and even newcomers who may approach the work from a different perspective or world view. While mentorship is explored in more detail in Chap. 3, the basic value proposition underpinning this book is that by listening in to stories of fellow travelers, you will both encounter new ways of approaching your work and by contrast develop the ability to reflect on your own style and approach with the goal of broadening your mental models and growing your behavioral and communicative repertoire.

As you read through the chapters, consider the practices, medical and communicative, of these doctors. Were their successes based on individual insight or team collaboration? How did they deal with conflicting interpretations of situations? Did they meet alternate analyses with curiosity or contempt? In new situations, such as the pandemic, did they simply try to manage, or did they create new procedures or routines that allowed them to not just survive the situation, but to flourish? How did they navigate the complex and uncertain environment of the ICU? What can you learn about successful (and unsuccessful) practices from their stories, insights, and personal experiences?

Leadership Requires Physicians to Navigate Competing Narratives Through Dialogue

Research makes clear that diverse, interdisciplinary teams make better decisions, but only when open communication is encouraged [12]. Organizational communication theorists recognize the power of dialogic communication to expand a leader's view of a situation by bringing together what are sometimes dramatically different perspectives [13, 14]. It is inevitable that patients and hospital employees will ascribe to divergent stories about what is happening on any given day; the job of the leader is to understand these varying narratives and to promote the aspects of their stories that they favor. Doing so requires two things: recognizing that in a real way perception is reality, whether you agree with it or not, and working to not see differing perspectives as oppositional, but rather as clues to a broader, more complex solution to a problem.

Making this happen in the ICU context requires a certain humility, the willingness to be expert but not always right, and a facility to ask good questions of people who think differently from you. Interestingly, the same interpersonal skills that make a good leader also work with patients: good listening, true presence without distractions, and a willingness to understand the situation from a perspective that can be radically different from one's own.

Next Steps in Using This Book

Becoming a more reflexive practitioner and seeking greater mastery of communication can pay off in many ways. But it is a tough path to walk because it requires you to pause and reflect on both current reality and your current communicative practice to create openings for change and improvement. Some steps you can take down this road look like this:

1. Get more data about how you show up to others. Ask trusted friends and colleagues how they see your strengths and weaknesses as a communicator, and listen to them.
2. Make explicit your assumptions and beliefs about your work environment, focusing on the stories you tell when people not associated with your organization ask you about your work. Identify what narratives you are repeating automatically out of habit, and decide if you want to continue to do so.
3. Related to the above, think deeply about the culture you would like to create—the ideal work environment—for you, your colleagues, and your patients. Once articulated, brainstorm small steps you could take immediately to begin constructing this vision of the future through your communication.
4. In team meetings and huddles, take a close look at agendas and how the meetings are organized. Determine if you make time for any reflection on group process, and experiment with reserving 5 minutes at the end of meetings to talk about how the meeting and work is organized. Ask for suggestions and try some out to see how things can improve.
5. Reflect on your own relationship with certainty, which is often shaped by your professional training. Create opportunities for colleagues and yourself to discuss things that are perhaps less certain and fixed than they appear and develop ways of speaking that encourage speculation and diversity of thought.
6. Take an inventory of communication practices you follow that focus on "delivering the message" but about which you have no clear indication that your intended message has been received. Shift your goal from delivering the message to checking for grasping of that message by the recipient.
7. Seek to create a culture of heedful interrelating and employee engagement in decision-making. Reflect on your socialization and orientation practices and the degree to which employees understand the nature of colleagues' work across departments. Reflect on your own leadership practice to ensure that employees understand the rationale behind decisions and, where possible, they can be involved in making them; people support what they help to create.

Mastering communication is a lifelong process for anyone who attempts it, but the upside is that any progress made has a positive impact both in and outside of work. The dynamic, fast-paced, life-and-death nature of the ICU puts unique pressure on doctors and others to keep up with the work, making little time or incentive to stop and reflect. This chapter has sought to illuminate both the benefits that can accrue through this kind of reflection and outlines some specific steps for incorporating reflexivity into your daily practice.

References

1. Watzlawick P, Beavin JH, Jackson DD. Pragmatics of human communication. New York: Norton; 1967.
2. Axley S. Managerial and organizational communication in terms of the conduit metaphor. Acad Manag Rev. 1984;9(3):428–37.
3. Feldman MS, March JG. Information in organizations as signal and symbol. Adm Sci Q. 1981;26:171–86.
4. Stohl C, Redding WC. Messages and message exchange processes. In: Jablin F, Putnam L, Roberts K, Porter L, editors. The handbook of organizational communication. Beverly Hills, CA: Sage; 1987.
5. Eisenberg EM, Mahar SE. Stop wasting words: leading through conscious communication. Charleston, SC: Advantage Media; 2019.
6. Craig R. Pragmatism in the field of communication theory. Commun Theory. 2007;17(2):125–45.
7. Giddens A. The constitution of society: outline of the theory of structuration. Berkley: University of California Press; 1984.
8. Taylor J, Van Every E. The emergent organization. Mahwah, NJ: Lawrence Erlbaum Associates; 2000.
9. Roscoe LA, Eisenberg EM, Forde C. The role of patients' stories in emergency medicine triage. Health Commun. 2016;31(9):1155–64.
10. Ellingson L. Communicating in the clinic. New York: Hampton Press; 2004.
11. Senge P. The fifth discipline: the art & Practice of the learning organization. New York: Doubleday/Currency; 2006.
12. Page S. The diversity bonus: how great teams pay off in the knowledge economy. Princeton: Princeton University Press; 2019.
13. Eisenberg E, Trethwey A, LeGreco M, Goodall HL. Organizational communication: balancing creativity and constraint. 8th ed. Boston: Bedford/St. Martin's; 2016.
14. Eisenberg E. The social construction of healthcare teams. In: Nemeth C, editor. Improving healthcare team communication: building on lessons from aviation and aerospace. Hampshire: Ashgate Publishing Ltd; 2008.

Chapter 3
Connecting People: How to Use the Book in a Mentoring Relationship

Diane Dennis ⓘ **and Kylie Julian**

In my walks, every man I meet is my superior in some way, and in that I learn from him

—Ralph Waldo Emerson

American quip writer Cullen Hightower once said, "A fool learns from his mistakes; a wise man learns from the mistakes of others", and this speaks to the heart of this book whereby an experienced group of people have taken the time to share their stories and expound their beliefs around the realities of functioning well as a doctor in the intensive care setting in the hope that others might benefit. These narratives are not just about mistakes. Hightower also said, "A true measure of your worth includes all of the benefits others have gained from your success". This book aspires to support trainees by placing them in a frame of preparation for their work in intensive care—preparation for success as much as for failure.

As alluded to in the previous chapter, the quotations found later within this book may be used by an individual as a basis for self-reflection—perhaps "walking a mile in their shoes" and experiencing meta-cognition of the events described. They may also be used in the context of a mentoring relationship, and this chapter explores that application. There is little hard evidence for mentoring in clinical medicine. Much of the literature about mentoring in medicine relates to academic medicine. Evidence in other contexts suggests that mentoring is associated with a range of positive outcomes, but overall effect sizes are small [1].

D. Dennis (✉)
Departments of Intensive Care and Physiotherapy, Sir Charles Gairdner Osborne Park Healthcare Group, Perth, WA, Australia
e-mail: diane.dennis@health.wa.gov.au

K. Julian
Department of Critical Care Medicine, Auckland City Hospital, Grafton, Auckland, New Zealand
e-mail: kyliej1@adhb.govt.nz

© The Author(s), under exclusive license to Springer Nature Switzerland AG 2025
D. Dennis et al. (eds.), *Contemplating the Role of an Intensive Care Doctor*,
https://doi.org/10.1007/978-3-031-92766-9_3

17

Speciality training imposes a series of goals, which in turn creates purpose. Mentoring provides an opportunity for independent goals that are personally and professionally relevant to be discussed. Asking how we relax into the role of an intensivist and reflect on our performance in that role without the external validation of feedback and assessment is important. How is success judged, once exams have been passed? How can success be defined in ways that are authentic to the values of the mentee? In his book *Mentoring 101*, John Maxwell [2] likens mentoring to growing a seed. He explains that while everyone has a unique seed of success within them, mentorship might be viewed as having someone identify and water that seed within a person. The mentoring relationship then works to help the seed to germinate and grow to reach its new potential. Within this construct, we can see that the contemporary model of mentoring is not about creating a "mini-me". It is instead about unlocking the potential to grow a new and unique model of a person that highlights utility of their strengths and minimises the impact of their shortcomings. Mentoring offers an opportunity to meet someone where they are at and then advance them in the direction they want to go to be the best version of themselves. It is also important to consider that being a mentor is not entirely altruistic—many find mentoring rewarding [3, 4]. The material in this book may therefore be used as foundational matter for mentoring relationships and conversations that examine and explore some of the issues surrounding the intensive care doctor as they work within the specialty.

There is increasing interest in formal college/society facilitated mentoring programmes in intensive care medicine. For example, the Australasian College of Intensive Care Medicine has a mentoring programme (www.cicm.org.au/Fellows/CICM-Mentoring-Programme), and the European Society of Intensive Care Medicine NEXT committee has reported on their experiences around setting up a mentorship programme [5]. Smaller regional mentoring programmes are also well established, such as the Auckland Regional Intensive Care Mentoring Programme for intensive care trainees in Auckland, New Zealand.

In academic medicine, minority groups are less likely to have a mentor than their peers, and women are less likely to have a mentor than men [6, 7]. Coordinated mentoring programmes, with an expectation of trainee participation, can work towards addressing inequity in intensive care medicine. Of note, compulsory or expected participation seems not to influence reported satisfaction with mentoring [8].

Modern approaches to mentoring suggest that there is benefit in having multiple mentors. This is not new, as it was certainly the case for the first mentee. Prior to departing Ithaca to fight in the Trojan war, Odysseus asked Mentor to guide and advise his infant son Telemachus. Disappointed in Mentor's performance, Athena, goddess of wisdom and war, took his form and assumed Mentor's role [9]. The quotations cited in this book were drawn from a wide group of intensivists—some working completely at the "coal face" of clinical life; others apportion part of their time to academia, research, or management. Some were close to retirement; others were earlier in their professional journey. The group therefore offers many perspectives and a diverse set of eyes through which to view and mentor a career in intensive care medicine. These will be valuable to mentees, experienced mentors, and those moving into a mentoring role.

In preparation for any mentoring connection, it is important from the outset for participants to define the "rules of engagement" for the relationship. The confidentiality of the mentoring relationship is based on mutual respect, and this must be affirmed at the beginning of the relationship, along with a discussion of the rare situations (concern for the safety of the mentee or of patients) that confidentiality would be broken. A clear discussion about conflicts of interest is also recommended, particularly when the mentee is in training. Any contribution of mentors to assessment must be based on clinical observation.

Mutual respect and the way this is demonstrated are also paramount to a successful mentoring partnership—being on time; being respectful of boundaries; active engagement and listening. We have emulated these rules in the way we have presented the data within this book. Our participants and any references to where and with whom they work have been deidentified. In terms of respect, there may be content within the scope of the quotations that you disagree with or find unlikely in the context of your own experiences as mentor or mentee. Know that they were considered a real concern for at least one of our participants and are thus normalised in that sense.

The establishment of "relevance" is another core consideration relating to the success of a mentoring relationship. Whether you agree or agree to disagree on the perspective presented within the quotations herein, the material discussed was extracted from transcripts of deep and considered conversations with experienced intensivists, and therefore its relevance cannot be overstated. As such, discussion and contemplation of these issues should both confirm, reinforce, and add validity to the relevance of the mentoring partnership between intensivist and intensivist trainee.

One of the important components of the mentoring relationship is for both parties to reflect on themselves at the beginning of their journey together. We have already explored elements of communication in Chap. 2, but there are other questions. How do I learn best? How do I prefer to give and receive feedback? Chap. 6 offers quotations and reflection points that will ask you to consider the traits of your personality and how they might align or differ from the person who has been quoted. How consistent are you? Do you consider yourself to have emotional intelligence? Are you assertive? What does assertion mean to you? How can you stand up or speak up with authenticity? Do you accept imperfection within yourself? Are you confident? What does confidence mean to you? How do you maintain confidence in the face of uncertainty? Are you able to deal with the uncertainty that often surrounds ICU care? As a mentee, have you considered these aspects of your personality? Are there gaps or concerns for you? Are you different altogether from the personalities described? And then, as the mentee shares their responses, do you, as a mentor, relate to any of the trepidations expressed around any of these domains? Arthur C. Benson, an English poet and writer, is quoted as saying that "People seldom refuse help if one offers it the right way". Can you, as a mentor, extend reassurance with tact, empathy, and genuine concern? Can you create a safe and non-judgmental space for your mentee? Can you share your stories? Can you reassure? Can you guide your mentee to consider other possibilities? Pondering these questions and reflecting on the comments shared in the chapter can help both mentee and mentor articulate their values.

The reason for mentorship should also be established early in the relationship because mentoring conversations are most rewarding when there is purpose—they should be conversations with intent and direction. In Chaps. 7 and 8, elements of the role of the intensivist and the environment in which they work are explored. Examining these aspects in detail, along with Chap. 6, will help mentee and mentor to define the expectations of their connection and set personal goals for mentorship. For example, is the focus going to be about navigating the environment? Is it going to be exploring things about the role itself and how that is perceived by others? Is it more about development of certain aspects of personality? Remember that the mentoring relationship is reciprocal: success requires an effective mentor and an engaged mentee. Outlining clear expectations, respect, and personal connection is essential. Mentor behaviours that contribute to success include making time to meet regularly and avoidance of conflicts of interest [4]. Effective mentees are open, are engaged in the process, and value their mentor's time [10]. The material within these chapters might help both parties to navigate this individualized path.

We all hold unconscious biases around ethnicity, gender, age, disability, and other factors that influence our perceptions and actions. The societal biases described in Chap. 9 seek to facilitate storytelling and sharing by both mentor and mentee of similar events within their career, with anecdotes of the outcomes, solutions, and learnings to be had. These experiences can also help shape the reciprocity that should define a mentoring relationship, in that both parties will learn from the connection, and each should bring a "we" not "me" approach to the union. The mentee can teach the mentor a lot about the top-down prejudices they have endured; the mentor might be reminded of what it was like to be in that position and may grow more empathy to bring to other working relationships. They may also suggest strategies that worked for them during their training. In addition, where there are shared lived experiences—two women might have faced the same misogynistic treatment—these will bond mentee and mentor each to the other for the journey moving forward.

These days we acknowledge the enormous and integral role that human factors play in error prevention within high-reliability organisations such as aviation, the armed forces, and healthcare. Of all the human factors, it is "communication" that is often cited as having critical importance in the context of safe patient-centred healthcare [11]. As such, we focus four chapters in Part 3 on examples within the domains of communication relevant to intensive care medicine: families, other doctors, dealing with children and parents, and the intensive care team. The mentor will have had significant lived experience in communicating within each of these realms, and because one of the tenants of a mentoring mindset is for the mentor to clear the mentees way, or at least have the mentee "fly with you a while", it is easy to imagine there will be many personal anecdotes spawned from the quotes provided that enable the personal growth of the mentee.

Of course, good communication also underpins a solid mentoring relationship, and so in parallel, the mentor/mentee couple should undertake to communicate with a high level of sophistication themselves. As the mentee shares their responses, mentors can reflect on how they relate to these questions. The mentor can create a safe and non-judgmental space for (or "that allows") the mentee to make their own conclusions. The mentoring conversation is a place where the expertise in communication essential for all intensivists can be modelled and practised. Conversations between mentors and mentees should be purposeful. They should provide opportunities to sit with silence, actively listen, and ask and be asked probing questions. There should be time set aside, patience, accepted permission to speak up, active listening, open questioning, genuine curiosity, and, in the end, a summary of the shared understanding.

In Chap. 15 and again in Chap. 17, we remind readers of the vulnerability of self-reflection. Those readers who began the book with some gaps and fragility may now begin to feel empowered. Those who have been confronted by things they had not prepared for may now feel discouraged. Both mentee and mentor might use this chapter to reflect on their engagement and enthusiasm within the relationship, recapping milestones, and reviewing goals. It is also a place where the mentor can be resourceful in providing introductions and opportunities to support the mentee where they are or take them to a higher level.

And so, both mentor and mentee may use the chapters that follow independently or together to foster growth of both themselves and each other. Mentoring relationships are places for reflection, goal setting, and solution finding. Mentoring models and develops a culture of collegial support and self-care, encourages the practice of critical reflection, contributes to the identification of personally and professionally important goals, and cultivates effective and meaningful work relationships. In closing, we hope that this field guide to intensive care medicine will contribute to mentorship within the specialty, because in the words of one of our respondents:

> To have a mentor… it's an incredibly important thing… I've learned a lot by watching her work. I think having a mentor is vital… not just practically but also in learning how to handle situations.

References

1. Eby LT, Allen TD, et al. Does mentoring matter? A multidisciplinary meta-analysis comparing mentored and non-mentored individuals. J Vocat Behav. 2008;72(2):254–67.
2. Maxwell JC. Mentoring 101: what every leader needs to know. Harper Collins; 2015.
3. Coates WC. Being a mentor: what's in it for me? Acad Emerg Med. 2012;19:92–7.
4. Jackson VA, Palepu A, et al. "Having the right chemistry": a qualitative study of mentoring in academic medicine. Acad Med. 2003;78:328–34.
5. De Rosa S, Battaglini D, Bennett V, Rodriguez-Ruiz E, Zaher AMS, Galarza L, Schaller SJ. NEXT committee of the ESICM. Key steps and suggestions for a promising approach to a critical care mentoring program. J Anesth Analg Crit Care. 2023;3(1):30. https://doi.org/10.1186/s44158-023-00116-4. PMID: 37644586; PMCID: PMC10464173

6. Ramanan RA, Taylor WC, et al. Mentoring and career preparation in internal medicine residency training. J Gen Intern Med. 2006;21:340–5.
7. Sambunjak D, Straus SE, et al. Mentoring in academic medicine: a systematic review. JAMA. 2006;296(9):1103–15.
8. Allen TD, Eby LT, et al. Mentorship behaviours and mentorship quality associated with formal mentoring programmes: closing the gap between research and practice. J Appl Psychol. 2006;91(3):567–78.
9. Homer. The Iliad. Translated by Robert Fagles, Penguin, 1991.
10. Straus SE, Johnson MO, et al. Characteristics of successful and failed mentoring relationships: a qualitative study across two academic health Centre. Acad Med. 2013;88:88–9.
11. Sameera V, Bindra A, Rath GP. Human errors and their prevention in healthcare. J Anaesthesiol Clin Pharmacol. 2021;37(3):328–35. https://doi.org/10.4103/joacp.JOACP_364_19. Epub 2021 Oct 12. PMID: 34759539; PMCID: PMC8562433

Chapter 4
Doing What's Right: How This Book Might Help to Prepare for Ethical Dilemmas in ICU

Melanie Jansen and Christopher Danbury ⓘ

> *We are speaking of no small matter, but how we ought to live.*
>
> —*Socrates*

The intensive care unit is a place where we, and our patients and their families, are regularly faced with high-stakes ethical decisions. We are often at the cutting edge of medical technology, both in our ICU therapies and in our role in supporting our subspecialty colleagues to care for their sickest patients. Life and death decisions are our everyday. In addition, we serve plural societies in which individual conceptions of quality of life and the perceptions of the burdens and benefits of therapies differ widely. Deciding on what the right course of action for a particular patient is can be harrowingly difficult.

Ethics is a prescriptive discipline that asks *what is the right thing to do*? Ethics is concerned with judgments of value. To say that we should take a particular course of action is to say that this course of action is better than others. We assign value and then we choose the path that has the most value. In intensive care practice, the process through which we choose which course of action to take is clinical reasoning. Clinical reasoning encompasses ethical reasoning, but we are generally less practised at making the ethical elements of our clinical reasoning explicit.

Every time you use an imperative word such as 'should', 'ought', and 'must', there is an ethical element to your rationale for why a particular action should be taken. You may reflect that you use these words all the time—*we should chart fluids for this patient; we ought to cease antibiotics; one of us must attend that trauma*

M. Jansen (✉)
Pediatric Intensive Care Unit, Qld Children's Hospital, South Brisbane, Australia

Clinical Ethics, Gold Coast Hospital and Health Service, Gold Coast, Australia

School of Historical and Philosophical Inquiry, University of Queensland, Brisbane, Australia

C. Danbury
Neurosciences Intensive Care Unit, University Hospital Southampton, Southampton, Hampshire, UK
e-mail: c.danbury@soton.ac.uk

D. Dennis et al. (eds.), *Contemplating the Role of an Intensive Care Doctor*, https://doi.org/10.1007/978-3-031-92766-9_4

23

call. This is because ethical claims are ubiquitous in the rationale for any action that may be taken in the future; therefore all clinical decisions are ethical decisions. The reason this is often not recognised is because, the majority of the time, the ethical claims we make in day-to-day practice are uncontroversial. A foundational ethical claim in the practice of medicine is that our purpose is to make treatment plans that will result in the best outcome for the patient. So, when we have a patient who needs to be kept nil by mouth, then the right thing to do is to chart intravenous fluids so they don't become dehydrated. We don't spell out the ethical premise (that we should do what is best for the patient) that underlies our conclusion (that we should chart fluids). This is because it is so obvious that it 'goes without saying'. It is a shared value among all healthcare practitioners.

Ethical tensions arise in cases where it is less clear what the 'best' course of action is. We rarely disagree with the ethical premise that we want to achieve the best outcome for the patient. But in some cases, this may be in conflict with other ethical obligations, such as the just distribution of resources or our obligation to ensure the well-being of ICU staff members. Commonly, we disagree on how to operationalise our desire to achieve the best outcome. For example, we may disagree on what the best outcome *is* for this patient; or we may question whether the patient really understands the consequences of their decision, especially when it is estimated that 80% of ICU patients lack capacity to decide for themselves. Similarly, we may question whether surrogate decision-makers (in jurisdictions that permit surrogates to make decisions) are making appropriate decisions, and if not, what is the threshold at which we should intervene? We may disagree on which treatment modality is the most likely to result in the best outcome. In complex patients who are cared for by multiple teams, the ownership of clinical decisions may be a source of ethical tension, and treatment modalities that require the cooperation of multiple specialties can require in-depth discussions. The clinical cannot be separated from the ethical.

So how do we make these decisions well? In the following sections, we discuss practical approaches to ensuring the ethical elements of our clinical decision-making are rigorous.

Ethical Principles in Intensive Care

The four principles of medical ethics [1], autonomy, beneficence, non-maleficence, and justice, are widely taught in medical schools. The authors argue that these principles are globally applicable. They also recognise that in clinical practice it is often difficult to perfectly uphold all these principles simultaneously and that clinicians need to weigh and prioritise these principles in the context of specific cases. Importantly, the four principles do not require adherence to a particular moral theory and so are appropriate for use in the plural societies that most of us serve. Some argue that principlism is, on its own, not sufficient for good ethical practice. There are other approaches to ethical reasoning. The Ethics of Care [2] draws our attention to elements of ethical practice that are outside of abstract moral reasoning. It has been described especially in relation to ensuring quality healthcare for vulnerable and marginalised groups. The Ethics of Care requires us to be attentive to who needs care; to take responsibility for providing care; to ensure we are competent to provide care; and to pay attention to whether we have meaningfully engaged the cared for. Narrative ethics is another approach to ethical analysis and decision making, where ethical insights and understanding are drawn from the narratives of patients, families, and clinicians. A comprehensive discussion of these approaches is outside the scope of this chapter, and it is worth noting that it is not necessary to choose one specific approach, as each can provide us with useful tools and insights for decision making in day to day practice. It is helpful to frame our thinking in such a way that recognises that in order to practise ethically, we need to engage in rigorous reasoning, while always paying close attention to the human stories of our patients. We need to understand the relationships within which they live and pay attention to how the relationships that we have with our patients, their families, and with our colleagues enable us to collaborate meaningfully to provide patient-centred care.

Multiple Ethical Obligations

In ICU we have multiple ethical obligations. Our primary obligation is to care for our patients and always strive to achieve the best outcome for them. We have an obligation, albeit a weaker one, to care for the patient's family and other loved ones, though some would argue this obligation is not a separate one, but an extension of our obligation to care for the patient. To achieve the best outcome for the patient, we need to understand who the patient is and what they value. What matters to them?

We are also obligated to ensure just stewardship of resources. This applies within our own units, where we prioritise and ration our bed spaces and staff according to need within our hospital. This 'bedside rationing' is often a more explicit part of day-to-day practice for those who practice in resource-limited settings. Regardless of the context in which we practice, as a specialty, we have an obligation to advise government and advocate for just stewardship of resources at a political level.

An ethical obligation that doesn't always immediately spring to mind when thinking about clinical ethics is our obligation to care for our clinical team. ICU is a physically and emotionally demanding job, whether you are a registered nurse, an allied healthcare professional, or a doctor. We have a responsibility to foster a positive workplace culture. With regard to ethical decision-making, we should strive to eliminate moral distress and never expect any staff member to participate in care that they feel is unconscionable.

While it is evident that ethical decision-making in ICU is complex and an enormous amount of medical and human information needs to be considered, you can't go far wrong if you consider these three things:

1. Do what is best for the patient, remembering that a decision to do nothing is still a decision with associated risks and benefits.
2. Do what is possible with the resources you have.
3. Don't expect anyone to carry out plans that they perceive to be unconscionable.

Procedural Justice—Accountability for Reasonableness in the ICU

The principles of procedural justice were developed by Norman Daniels for use in healthcare rationing decisions [3]. Daniels developed these principles as, after many years of research and teaching about rationing, he and others had failed to elucidate principles that everyone agreed on for how to ration healthcare resources. He concludes that exactly how to ration resources is something 'about which reasonable people may disagree'. In light of this, he advocates shifting our focus to *how* we make the decision. If our decision process has been just, then we can agree that the decision is *legitimate*, even if all people don't agree with the final decision in a particular case. Daniels also points out that over time, if we adhere to the principles of just decision-making, this will foster ongoing learning and reflection on the ethics that inform our decisions.

The principles of procedural justice are as follows:

1. Transparency—the rationale for decisions must be clearly stated and available to all who have a stake in the decision.
2. Relevance—the rationale must be reasoned and must only include considerations that are relevant to the situation at hand.
3. Review and appeal—there must be a mechanism for appeal and review of decisions.
4. Enforcement—there must be a mechanism to ensure that the above principles are upheld.

These principles were discussed widely during the COVID-19 pandemic and have since been applied to other clinical contexts outside of rationing decisions. Because we serve plural societies, and because medicine and the humans it cares for are complex, there is rarely a single 'best' solution to a given clinical problem. Almost every case in medicine is something 'about which reasonable people may disagree'. That there are many ways to 'skin a cat' is an idiom often invoked by intensivists when discussing day to day ICU practice.

In addition, ICU medicine is a team sport. All of our decision-making is collaborative, and there are multiple stakeholders for clinical decisions—the patient, their family, and the multidisciplinary team, both within and outside of ICU. All ICU patients are co-managed by at least one other specialty team. Even in closed ICUs, there are clinical decisions, such as whether to take a surgical patient back to theatre, that remain the remit of the specialty team. Importantly, delivery of high-quality intensive care requires a large multidisciplinary team of doctors, nurses, and allied healthcare professionals. Department cohesion will be higher if all team members understand the rationale for the management plans that they are carrying out. Moral distress—the feeling that arises when you feel your ability to do the right thing is constrained—has been well described in nursing staff and junior doctors. Understanding the rationale for clinical decisions, and knowing that decisions were made thoughtfully and comprehensively, may help to alleviate this.

Decision-Making Processes in ICU

So What Does a Just Decision-Making Process in ICU Look Like?

Of course, there are many ways to skin a cat, but we suggest the following process. The higher the stakes of the decision, the more exhaustive and comprehensive these steps should be. Depending on urgency, these steps can be pragmatically truncated. The steps in this suggested process have been modified from previous research on complex decision-making in intensive care [4], and much of the explanatory information is drawn from a paper on the critical appraisal of ethics literature [5]. We will refer to the following vignette:

AB is a 25-year-old man, who was involved in a high-speed road traffic collision (RTC). The driver of a car, he was 'T-boned' by another vehicle.

The RTC caused AB to suffer significant injuries. He was extracted from his car by the emergency services and was intubated and ventilated at the scene by the attending Helicopter Emergency Medical Service (HEMS) doctor. Following the helicopter transfer to the regional Major Trauma Centre, AB was assessed in the Emergency Department (ED) by the Trauma team. Following a trauma CT of the head, chest, abdo, and pelvis, he was diagnosed with the following injuries: traumatic brain injury (TBI) consisting of traumatic right frontal subarachnoid haemorrhage with contrecoup injury, bilateral pneumothoraces, multiple rib fractures bilaterally, small bowel contusion, grade 2 laceration of spleen, and a compound fracture of his left tibia and fibula. His immediate life-threatening injury was the TBI. He had intercostal catheters sited in the pneumothoraces, and his leg was cleaned but not fixed due to the TBI. His abdominal injuries were treated conservatively, and TPN was recommended to minimise stress to the gastrointestinal tract.

AB was admitted to the neuroscience/trauma ICU following his primary and secondary surveys in the ED. An intracranial pressure monitor was sited, and medical management of his intracranial pressure (ICP) was commenced.

At this point, his family arrived in the hospital, and the duty ICU consultant discussed A's management with his family. His parents were healthcare professionals, although not in trauma-related fields. His three siblings were also present, none of whom had followed their parents into healthcare.

The life-threatening nature of the TBI was raised as were possible treatment options should the medical management be insufficient to control AB's ICP. Options discussed were an extraventricular drain (EVD) and decompressive crainiectomy. EVD involves putting a thin plastic tube into the ventricles of the brain to allow cerebrospinal fluid (CSF) to be drained, thus reducing the pressure within the skull. Decompressive craniectomy involves removing part of the skull to allow the brain to swell into that area, again minimising the increase in ICP. The RESCUE-icp study was discussed as this showed that "At 6 months, decompressive craniectomy in patients with traumatic brain injury and refractory intracranial hypertension resulted in lower mortality and higher rates of vegetative state, lower severe disability, and upper severe disability than medical care. The rates of moderate disability and good recovery were similar in the two groups".

The immediate response from AB's parents was that he would not want to live with a severe brain injury and that he would not want a decompressive craniectomy. AB's siblings were not as certain as their parents.

Over the next 36 hours, it was necessary to site an EVD and AB's ICP looked to be slowly increasing.

Several further discussions occurred with the family about AB's wishes and preferences in the days following admission to ICU. These discussions included various senior members of the ICU and neurosurgical teams. These discussions were to ensure that AB's wishes and preferences were properly understood and respected. Over this time, the parents became less certain about their initial, instinctive opinion of AB's views. Seventy-two hours after admission, it was agreed that actually AB would probably want the increased chance of surviving, even if that meant an increased chance of survival with severe brain injury.

At 120 h (5 days) following admission, AB went for a decompressive craniectomy due to failure of medical management.

One hundred twenty hours after decompressive craniectomy, medical management was weaned over a number of days.

> *AB's motor score of his GCS was M6.*

> *Six months following admission, AB had a left sided weakness of both arm and leg. He needed help with activities of daily living, but was very grateful for all the treatment, including the decompressive craniectomy.*

Identify Stakeholders

Ensure you have consulted with and included everyone who may have a stake in the situation: the patient and/or their surrogate decision-maker/s; other family members/friends with an interest in the patient's welfare; the ICU multidisciplinary team; relevant subspecialty teams; social workers; pastoral care practitioners; and cultural support workers. This list is not exhaustive.

Information Gathering

In any clinical case, we gather as much detailed medical information as we can. In the case of AB, we want to know details such as the mechanism of injury, the GCS at the scene, other injuries sustained, imaging and other findings from the trauma assessments, and much more. This is so we can prioritise his clinical management, have clues on what to expect in the coming days, and have as much prognostic information as possible. This is a process that most intensivists are intimately familiar with.

The other imperative information is the human understanding. The central human is, of course, the patient. Who is AB? Who are his closest family and friends? What did AB like to do with his time? What did he value? One of the key ways that humans understand themselves and their place in the world is through narrative. Be curious about the story of the patient and their family. What *matters* for them? Ask the family to show you photos or videos of their family member when they were well. In AB's case, his family were initially not in total alignment about what they thought his wishes would be. Patients and families often need time and multiple conversations to work out exactly how much value they place on things like physical mobility and different dimensions of cognitive and relational capacity. They need time and thoughtful conversation with the healthcare team and other loved ones to work out what degree and type of uncertainty they can tolerate and what their best and worst case scenarios are, among other things. Does AB's family understand what 'upper severe' disability would really be like on a day-to-day basis? Would AB want a chance at living with good function and be happy to take the risk of ending up with significant disability, or would living with any degree of disability be 'a fate worse than death' for him?

The other humans involved in the decision are the clinical stakeholders. We all bring our prior experiences, biases, and emotions to every situation. Ethical tension and moral distress are very emotive. This is appropriate—we feel strong emotions about things that matter. Acknowledging and addressing emotions in high stakes, group decision-making is important for two key reasons. (1) Strong emotions often highlight important tensions in a case—discussing the thoughts and reasons underlying emotions can illuminate key aspects of a case, which, once recognised, can then be thoughtfully addressed and incorporated into the rationale for the clinical management. (2) If we attempt to 'leave the emotions out of it' and make 'objective' decisions, the emotions will instead implicitly and, possibly inappropriately, impact the group dynamics and decision-making. This may then breed moral distress and a lack of faith in the decisions being made.

Clarification of Questions and Definitions of Important Terms

Once we have gathered comprehensive information, we should be clear what the ethical question is that we are trying to answer. Imagine that on day 1 of admission, when AB's ICP was well controlled on first-tier therapy, his family is advocating for withdrawal of life sustaining therapy due to their assertion that he would not want to live with disability. The ethical question then may be *is it reasonable to withdraw LST in this case?* Or we could imagine the opposite problem—that AB has refractory intracranial hypertension and progresses to brain death. His family believes that he may still recover and requests continuing ventilation for at least 3 weeks to wait for recovery. The ethical question then may be *is it reasonable to acquiesce to the family's request and continue ventilation for 3 weeks?* Having a clear question around which to anchor the discussion helps the team to remain focused on the key problem and develop a practical solution.

Defining the terms we use in any discussion is important. For example, in any clinical guideline that is written, the first task is to define the terms used. When we say that sepsis is *life-threatening organ dysfunction associated with a dysregulated host response to infection*, we then define what 'life-threatening organ dysfunction' is. Likewise, if someone says that AB is not likely to have good quality of life if he has a decompressive craniectomy, we should then explore what they think AB would consider a good quality of life. In fact, one of the criticisms of the RESCUE-icp trial was that it was initially reported as a positive trial because it increased the number of survivors with a 'good' neurological outcome. The definition of 'good' was 'upper severe disability', in contrast to the DECRA trial [6, 7] which designated a 'good' outcome as 'moderate' disability.

Analysis of Arguments

Once we have gathered comprehensive information, we must then analyse the arguments for and against possible clinical plans. We use the word 'argument' in the philosophical sense, meaning 'a set of reasons that justifies a position'. We could also call it a 'rationale'. To critically analyse arguments, we must first understand how arguments are structured.

Arguments are made up of premises and conclusions. Premises are things we take to be true. Conclusions are drawn by reasoning from the premises. You may disagree with an argument for two reasons. Either you think the premises are untrue, or the reasoning from the premises to the conclusion is not valid. For example, in the case of AB, his parents initially said they did not want him to have a decompressive craniectomy as he would definitely not want to live with any disability. Their argument would be structured in the following way:

Premise 1: We should make a decision that respects AB's wishes.
Premise 2: AB would not want to live with any degree of disability.
Premise 3: Decompressive craniectomy will increase the chances of AB living with disability.
Therefore,
Conclusion: We do not consent to AB having a decompressive craniectomy.

AB's siblings disagree with his parents because they are not so sure that Premise 2 is true. The task, then, is to explore their thoughts about AB's values and discuss in more detail what is really important to him functionally and whether it is really true that he would not want to live with 'any' degree of disability, or if actually he would rather be alive with some hemiplegia, as long as he can still self-mobilise, and have good cognitive capacity.

When questioning the truth of the premises of an argument, it is also useful to identify whether the premise is a factual claim or a value claim, as this will help to explore its veracity appropriately. In the above argument, Premise 1 is a value claim (AB's parents are saying that they 'should' do something); and Premise 2 and 3 are factual claims. Premise 2 is an experiential fact, i.e. we can only explore the truth of this claim by questioning reported personal experience. In the ICU this is often (as described above) done by exploring the 'best guess' of the surrogate decision-maker. Premise 3 is an empirical fact, i.e. one that can be supported or nullified by scientific research. If you disagreed with this premise, you would need to find robust scientific research to support your claim.

An example of invalid reasoning could be as follows: a colleague who had one family meeting with AB's family is handing over to you. *When I spoke with AB's family, they said that he is a very risk-averse person. Because decompressive craniectomy has a high risk of resulting in disabled survivors, I don't think this will be something they will consent to.* In this case the argument may be structured in the following way:

Premise 1: Decompressive craniectomy increases the chance of surviving TBI with disability.
Premise 2: AB's parents state that AB is a risk-averse person.
Therefore,
Conclusion: They are unlikely to consent to decompressive craniectomy.

In this case, even if Premise 1 and 2 are true, it may not necessarily follow that AB's parents are unlikely to consent to a decompressive craniectomy—so it is the reasoning that is being questioned. It would be important to explore fully what they meant when they said that AB is 'risk-averse'. The conclusion that they are unlikely to consent to decompressive craniectomy may even be true, but their decision may not be solely based on their perception of his risk-averseness.

Development and Documentation of Plan

Once the arguments for and against different possible plans have been thoroughly explored, the chosen plan should be documented, along with the explicit rationale underlying that plan. A common gripe from hospital legal services is that clinical reasoning is not well documented. Clearly documenting the decision-making process and rationale is medicolegally protective.

Review

All complex decisions should be reviewed. In most departments this would be done at departmental meetings such as morbidity and mortality meetings or as part of reflective discussions or debriefs for difficult cases.

Summary and Food for Thought

What is the right thing to do? This is a question that, as intensive care clinicians, we should never stop asking ourselves. The immensity of the decisions we are faced with, the complexity of the human and medical information that we must synthesize and work through, can feel overwhelming. Always remember that ICU is a team sport and that the ethical decision-making we do in ICU medicine is no exception. Take some time, be inclusive and comprehensive in what you consider, seek clarity, think through the reasons carefully, and listen to those who challenge you. Do what is best for the patient, do what you can with the resources you have, and make sure the team can deliver the care with a good conscience, and you can't go far wrong.

References

1. Beauchamp TL, Childress JF. Principles of medical ethics. Oxford University Press; 2001.
2. Barns KJE, Peachey L. (Girrimay/Djirribal), Seeking a voice: the inadequacy of the "four principles" and the need for care ethics in the provision of health care to vulnerable populations. Med J Aust. 2024;221(1):25–8. https://doi.org/10.5694/mja2.52349.
3. Daniels N. Accountability for reasonableness. BMJ. 2000;321(7272):1300–1. https://doi.org/10.1136/bmj.321.7272.1300.
4. Jansen M, Moynihan KM, Taylor LS, Basu S. Complex decision-making in Pediatric intensive care: a discussion paper and suggested model. Bioeth Inq. 2024; https://doi.org/10.1007/s11673-024-10381-9. Online ahead of print.
5. Jansen M, Ellerton P. How to read an ethics paper. J Med Ethics. 2018;44(12):810–3. https://doi.org/10.1136/medethics-2018-104997. Epub 2018 Aug 22
6. Hutchinson PJ, Kolias AG, Timofeev IS, Corteen EA, Czosnyka M, Timothy J, Anderson I, et al. Trial of Decompressive Craniectomy for traumatic intracranial hypertension. N Engl J Med. 2016;375:1119–30.
7. Cooper DJ, Rosenfeld JV, Murray L, Arabi M, Davies AR, D'Urso P, Kossmann T, et al. Decompressive Craniectomy in diffuse traumatic brain injury. N Engl J Med. 2011;364:1493–502.

Chapter 5
Balancing Insight with Serenity: How to Use the Book to Self-Reflect But Not Ruminate

Adam van Heerden

> *As for the future, your task is not to foresee it, but to enable it.*
>
> —*Antoine de Saint Exupery*

Memory has the capacity to take us deep into our personal and collective history, but the evolutionary function of the memory system is inherently *prospective*. We remember in order to prepare for a contingent but potentially controllable future. Emergent from the memorial system is the striking ability for future oriented imaginings or what is whimsically referred to as future mental time travel [1]. We can gaze into the crystal ball and plant ourselves in an imagined future scenario in our mind's eye.

Future-oriented mental time travel may have led to detention in high school, but the degree to which we can harness this ability to imagine and plan for challenging future scenarios will increase our preparedness and adaptability to face these (or similar) scenarios when they arise. Further, the extent to which we can predict the nature of future decisions actually reshapes the memory system to pay attention to salient information that may be useful in making those very decisions [2]. Such memory-based planning and anticipatory tendencies can be traced back hundreds of thousands of years and have played a significant role in the collective survival of our ancestors. In a similar vein, we hope that by actively imagining and preparing for future contingencies, the reader will not only survive but thrive in the ICU context.

However, all superpowers have their shadow side, and future-oriented self-reflection is no exception. Gazing too intently into the crystal ball has the potential to become a fixation that traps the gazer in the realms of rumination and worry. If this spell is cast, their thought patterns will become passive and perseverate, dominated by the doom and gloom of a seemingly uncontrollable future, or repetitively anchored to notions of failure and self-criticism.

A. van Heerden (✉)
Inner Spark Psychology, Naarm, Melbourne, Australia

© The Author(s), under exclusive license to Springer Nature
Switzerland AG 2025
D. Dennis et al. (eds.), *Contemplating the Role of an Intensive Care Doctor*,
https://doi.org/10.1007/978-3-031-92766-9_5

Antidote 1: Realize Your Problems Are Not Unique

This is the inverse intention of this book, which is meant to cultivate hope and psychologically prepare the intensivist for a successful career. By immersing themselves in the stories and wisdom of intensivists who have already traversed the path, the reader is invited into the fellowship of intensive care specialists and reminded that they are not alone in the challenges that arise. This is the first antidote to ward off the spell of rumination and worry. In the no-nonsense words of Mark Manson [3], "Realize that your problems are not special or unique, that you are not special and unique." While this advice may appear harsh and even a little rude, Manson sees this as "good news. Because it means that you will never ever have to suffer alone."

It would be terrifying if our problems were novel because the onus would be entirely upon us to generate an equally novel solution. Rather, we can rely on the experience of others who have gone before us and reap practical advice from their failures and successes. Medical students spend endless hours poring over past case studies, in the hope that this information will be instructive for the patients they come to treat. While no two patients are entirely alike, the tradition of case studies (or the "doctrine of precedent" in law), suggests that knowledge can be applied across similar cases. Thus, the aspiring intensivist can enter their specialty with the confidence that the vast majority of problems that arise have been encountered and overcome by their predecessors.

Beyond receiving practical guidance from the experience of others, recognizing that our problems are not unique fosters a sense of belonging and shared experience [4]. All humans make mistakes and undergo difficulty. Thus, framing our own challenges as a form of common humanity buffers against isolation and shame and is a key component of self-compassion [5].

The alternative is to feel defective and allow our flaws to threaten our sense of belonging—a fundamental human need. While contemplating the quotations throughout this book, the reader is invited to frame their own challenges as a normal part of being human and as part and parcel of the intensive care specialty. In doing so, the reader is welcomed into the broader community of intensive care specialists and takes their place within a long-standing discipline that strives for compassion toward others, as well as a healthy dose of self-compassion.

Antidote 2: Think Specific

Aside from framing our challenges and flaws as a part of a common humanity, the second antidote to depressive rumination requires a specific type of thinking. Depressive rumination is characterized by over-generalized verbal-analytical thinking that centers on negative social comparison, the repetitive questioning of *why* an adverse event occurred, and a focus on the "catastrophic" consequences. This type of cognition is decontextualized and involves global and immutable valuations of self and others. For example, "I'm a failure," rather than "I made a mistake." It focuses on the general gist of an action or event but lacks the specificity to convey nuance [6]. Such global mental representations and overgeneralized memory of adverse events amplify emotional reactivity [7] and are implicated in increased risk of depression [8].

By contrast, concrete and specific thinking that is process-focused and imagery-based mitigates these injurious effects on mood and cognition, despite an equivalent level of self-referential focus [9]. For instance, participants who were asked to visually imagine a challenging emotional scenario in as much detail as possible and then presented with an insoluble problem-solving task displayed far less negative affect than those asked to think abstractly about the same scenario [6]. This experiment suggests that concrete and specific thinking is both a trainable and effective buffer against the detrimental effects of depressive rumination.

Therefore, when reflecting on the challenging scenarios outlined in this book, we urge the reader to focus on *how* an adverse event occurred by paying careful attention to the details and context of each specific situation. If it feels psychologically safe to do so, we invite the reader to imagine each scenario as vividly and in as much detail as possible, as if a movie were screening in their mind's eye. Such specific and concrete thinking will support the reader to gain maximum insight from their reflections on how they may relate to challenging events while simultaneously shielding them from the possibility of engaging in over-generalized negative self-attributions.

Antidote 3: It's All in the Timing

Besides being strategic about the type of thinking, it's equally important to consider the timing when addressing challenging future scenarios in intensive care. There is a well-known psychological intervention called "Worry Time," in which one is asked to carve out a designated time to contend with their worries, rather than being at the whim of their worries throughout the day. During the allocated "Worry Time," individuals confront their worries directly, either by problem-solving or by practicing acceptance of situations beyond their control. Paradoxically, setting aside time to worry productively reduces the overall time spent worrying and may contribute to decreased stress levels.

However, the "Worry Time" technique must be used carefully to be effective. To this end, psychologists have developed a number of guidelines, some of which may be instructive for our purposes here. Firstly, it is critical to set a 15–30-minute time limit to safeguard against open-ended worrying. "Worry Time" is designed to be a focused and productive activity that directly addresses one's troubles. Similarly, it may be useful to demarcate a clear time-block when contemplating some of the more challenging scenarios in this book. Moreover, as with "Worry Time," it is important to consider the time of day one reflects on the difficult scenarios that may arise in the intensive care specialty. Since impaired attentional control is associated with increased and persistent rumination [10], one is advised to engage in self-reflection when they have adequate cognitive and attentional resources at their disposal. This leads to the final guideline—it is crucial to transition out of the allotted self-reflection time. An enjoyable transitional activity like calling a friend or going for a walk may be useful in helping the reader mindfully terminate their self-reflection and redirect their attention elsewhere.

The "Worry Time" intervention indicates the utility of tackling our concerns voluntarily and strategically. By engaging in the technique, the individual not only addresses their worries productively but also signals to themselves that their worries need not control them. Rather, they have the capacity to directly face their worries and relate to them in a wise manner.

Antidote 4: Be Proactive

By being proactive in this manner, one deviates from the underlying schematic structure of rumination and worry. Namely, one cultivates the belief that one's environment can be influenced and managed by planful actions. If you are reading this book, the chances are that you already exhibit some proactive personality traits. People with a proactive personality tend to shape rather than passively accept their environment [11]. They consistently engage in proactive behaviors to prepare for the future and improve their circumstances, which in turn leads to increased optimism and hope.

New research suggests that weekly future optimism—actively envisioning and preparing for one's future—is positively related to weekly subjective well-being [12]. By reflecting on and preparing for the future, one gets a better handle on the nature of potential future challenges and how one might adaptively respond. In doing so, the future becomes more predictable and less anxiety provoking. There is no denying that intensive care specialists encounter intractable situations, but with a proactive and planful attitude, the reader is well placed to face any challenge that arises.

Antidote 5: Remember Your "Why"

It is important to note that the current book includes reflections on the challenges *and* triumphs of intensive care clinicians. The picture would not be complete with a binary focus on one or the other, as the reality of the intensive care specialty encompasses both success and failure, fatigue and fulfillment, and loss and recovery. Due to an adaptive evolutionary bias, danger and negativity are more salient to the human mind than positively valanced emotions [13]. While this may have contributed to our survival, it means we must actively nurture positive emotionality.

Within the context of this book, the reader is encouraged not to exclusively focus on the quotations that highlight difficult future scenarios. Linger a while on the positively valanced reflections, and let them be a portal to your own motivations for practicing intensive care medicine. What possibilities might exist for the compassion and care you extend to a patient and their family? What qualities do you admire in the clinicians you are reading about? What first interested you in intensive care, and what are your hopes for your future career? Remember your "why" and let it fortify you. In the words of Viktor Frankl [14], "Those who have a 'why' to live, can bear with almost any 'how'."

Research on the experience of early medical students revealed human connection as the primary "why" that allowed them to bear the frustrations of medical school. Despite the overwhelming stressors and internal conflicts about being a doctor, relationships with peers, and especially the idealized connection with one's future patients, made the struggle worthwhile. As one medical student writes [15]: "What I love about medical school is this idea in my mind that hopefully someday soon I will be working with real people, not just the fake ones I read about in vignettes. Shaking their hands, smiling, treating, and in some cases grieving. *What I love about medical school is the idea that one day I'll be dealing with the issues of humanity and that no matter how small I may be, I will have some small part to play in others' lives while I'm here.*"

This is the "why" that overcomes almost any "how"—the existential "why" that replenishes and might fortify the reader in times of difficulty. Notice the common humanity in the excerpt above. The medical student simply wishes to play their part in the grand story of humanity. Through engaging with the current book, the reader is encouraged to reflect on their own "why" as a means of cultivating hope and motivation for their career as an intensive care specialist. The reader is once again welcomed into the broader community of medical practitioners and intensive care specialists, in particular. They are asked to take their place in the chain of clinicians that aspire to heal and do no harm to the suffering patients that come before them. The hope is that these five antidotes support the aspiring intensivist to balance insight with serenity and gaze into the crystal ball in a wise manner that recognizes that neither they nor their patients need ever suffer alone.

References

1. Klein SB. The complex act of projecting oneself into the future. WIREs Cognitive Sci. 2013;4(1):63–79. https://doi.org/10.1002/wcs.1210.
2. Klein SB, Cosmides L, Tooby J, Chance S. Decisions and the evolution of memory: multiple systems, multiple functions. Psychol Rev. 2002;109(2):306–29.
3. Manson M. The subtle art of not giving a F*ck: a counterintuitive approach to living a good life. Harper One; 2016.
4. Tajfel H, Turner JC. An integrative theory of intergroup conflict. In: Austin WG, Worchel S, editors. The social psychology of intergroup relations. Monterey: Brooks/Cole; 1979. p. 33–7.
5. Neff KD. Self-compassion: an alternative conceptualization of a healthy attitude toward oneself. Self Identity. 2003;2:85–101.

6. Watkins E, Moberly NJ, Moulds ML. Processing mode causally influences emotional reactivity: distinct effects of abstract versus concrete construal on emotional response. Emotion. 2008;8(3):364–78. https://doi.org/10.1037/1528-3542.8.3.
7. Wenzlaff RM, Grozier SA. Depression and the magnification of failure. J Abnorm Psychol. 1988;97:90–3.
8. Williams JMG, Barnhofer T, Crane C, Hermans D, Raes F, Watkins E, et al. Autobiographical memory specificity and emotional disorder. Psychol Bull. 2007;133(1):122–48.
9. Rimes KA, Watkins E. The effects of self-focused rumination on global negative self-judgements in depression. Behav Res Ther. 2005;43:1673–81.
10. Caulfield MK, Hallion LS. Impaired disengagement from worry: dissociating the impacts of valence and internally-directed attention. Behav Res Ther. 2023;161:Article 104242. https://doi.org/10.1016/j.brat.2022.104242.
11. Fuller JBJ, Marler LE. Change driven by nature: a meta-analytic review of the proactive personality literature. J Vocat Behav. 2009;75(3):329–45. https://doi.org/10.1016/j.jvb.2009.05.008.
12. Wang S, Tu Y, Zhao T, Yang Y. Focusing on the past, present, or future? Why proactive personality increases weekly subjective Well-being. J Happiness Stud. 2022;23(5):1543–60. https://doi.org/10.1007/s10902-021-00461-7.
13. Baumeister RF, Finkenauer C, Vohs KD. Bad is stronger than good. Rev Gen Psychol. 2001;5(4):323–70. https://doi.org/10.1037/1089-2680.5.4.323.
14. Frankl VE. Man's search for meaning (A. J. P. Legg, trans.). Beacon Press. 2006.(Original work published 1946).
15. MacArthur KR, Sikorski J. A qualitative analysis of the coping reservoir model of pre-clinical medical student Well-being: human connection as making it 'worth it'. BMC Med Educ. 2020;20(1):157. https://doi.org/10.1186/s12909-020-02067-8.

Part II
Swimming Lessons

Foreword: How to Swim, One Stroke at a Time

Michael Ruppe

> I actually love swimming, but I just hate jumping in the water. (Natalie Coughlin)

Intensive care unit doctor. Intensivist. Intense. To thrive in this career is to confidently accept the role of lifeguard, looking out over the choppy water as the hurricane approaches. In the next several chapters, we will peel back the layers to reveal the person behind the ICU career. We start with the ICU mindset; what makes a doctor in training seek out the most critically ill patients and face the most emotional and fearful moments in a family's life? What human qualities align with the demands of a day in the ICU? Throughout a career, what personality traits make the difference between surviving and thriving?

ICU doctors must swim headfirst through the ever-changing forces of nature. They are called on to assume countless roles; team leader, diplomat, proceduralist, researcher and counsellor, to name a few. We will explore how an ICU career matures, block by block and role by role. Some intensivists excel in compassionately guiding families through end-of-life decisions. Others thrive on the mental challenges inherent in multi-organ dysfunction and extremes of pathophysiology. Yet every ICU doctor needs to remain nimble; placing a life-saving central line one minute can progress to mediating a tense discussion amongst consulting clinical teams the next. The list goes on and on.

As we dive deeper into the ICU doctor's life, we will examine the environment in which they work. ICU's are fitted with all of the essentials to combat these extremes of illness. The technology and capabilities are ever-changing. The pace of drug development, technological upgrades or even artificial intelligence and machine learning requires today's intensivist to perpetually adopt new sciences and new ways to improve outcomes.

Intensivists also need strength and endurance to stay afloat during the catastrophic floods. We must also address the realities of burnout, the emotional toll on both staff and families, the 24-hour nature of the job and the inevitability of death. Additionally, we will confront biases in the care that we provide and the career that we have chosen. As intensivists in a modern era, we are acutely impacted by the challenges of race and class. We strive for equity while practicing within the confines of fiscal responsibility and we persevere often against a backdrop of ageism, sexism and discrimination.

Finally, we will explore society's perception of the ICU doctor's career, a topic that has never been more scrutinized than during the COVID-19 pandemic. Today's ICU is a place that routinely and successfully treats patients with conditions that were fatal only a few decades ago [1, 2]. This sobering yet inspiring reality can make the ICU seem like a surreal battleground with the ICU doctor assuming the role of Admiral.

References

1. Zimmerman JE, Kramer AA, Knaus WA. Changes in hospital mortality for United States intensive care unit admissions from 1988 to 2012. Crit Care. 2013;17(2):R81. https://doi.org/10.1186/cc12695. PMID: 23622086; PMCID: PMC4057290.
2. van Breugel JMM, Niemeyer MJS, Houwert RM, Groenwold RHH, Leenen LPH, van Wessem KJP. Global changes in mortality rates in polytrauma patients admitted to the ICU-a systematic review. World J Emerg Surg. 2020;15(1):55. https://doi.org/10.1186/s13017-020-00330-3. PMID: 32998744; PMCID: PMC7526208.

Chapter 6
Can You Swim? Contemplating Your Personality

Carl Horsley

Knowing yourself is the beginning of all wisdom

—Aristotle

Intensive care is one of the most challenging areas in healthcare. It involves high stakes, time-critical decision-making, a huge body of relevant knowledge, and the significant emotional demands that come from caring for the critically ill. Intensive care therefore places significant personal demands on those who choose to work there.

This chapter asks readers to contemplate various aspects of intensive care and explore how our practice is shaped by the individual perspectives and differences we bring to the work. The aim is not to describe some 'ideal' to aspire to, but rather it is an opportunity to understand ourselves better. By doing so, we see how our different personalities, experiences, and values give different answers to the question "What kind of intensivist will I be?"

Surfing the Chaos or Controlled Precision?

There's almost a spectrum, where anaesthetists are at one end where they want a very controlled environment that is extremely predictable, and emergency physicians are at the other end where they just want chaos. The intensivist has to be somewhere in the middle, and you can kind of see people who are more down the anaesthetist side, like more down the fastidious OCD (Obsessive Compulsive Disorder) side, where they just get so put out by unexpected emergencies that it is untenable. And then at the other end, you've got people who are so happy working in a less controlled environment that they don't

C. Horsley (✉)
Middlemore Hospital, Auckland, New Zealand
e-mail: Carl.Horsley@cmdhb.org.nz

© The Author(s), under exclusive license to Springer Nature Switzerland AG 2025
D. Dennis et al. (eds.), *Contemplating the Role of an Intensive Care Doctor*,
https://doi.org/10.1007/978-3-031-92766-9_6

fastidiously check all the things that we routinely do in the ICU. So, I think that you have to be able to balance those competing demands.

- Whether you have heard this description before or not, consider it now. Where do you think that you fit across this scale of needing a controlled environment to function well? What is it like for you when you can't practice this way?
- How comfortable are you when dealing with situations which pull your attention in multiple directions? What strategies have you developed or observed in others?
- How do you manage the trade-off of trying to deal with multiple competing demands yet still practice safely? What situations make it more difficult to manage?
- Have you experienced situations where something important was missed because the ICU was so busy? How did it feel when you realised?
- Needing to have a sense of control can sometimes lead people to micromanage situations. Have you ever been on the receiving end of this approach? How did it make you feel?

Scanning the Horizon

Most of us are 'control freak', 'worst-case-scenario' people, and so most of us like to plan for the worst, and if it's better, we are excited… I think as a whole, all of us in the intensive care, at least in our group, are very much like that … 'knowing what's going to happen and having that plan'.

- A reportedly common trait of the intensivist is the ability to anticipate possible trajectories for the patient. Forward planning with clear articulation of those plans is a common strategy. Think of a time when an intensivist went through a catalogue of potential future events with you and the appropriate actions to be taken in response to those events. What were the positive and negative impacts on your ongoing management of that patient?
- Consider a time you were surprised by a patient's course. What were your expectations before the event occurred, and what was it that made it so surprising?
- How easy do you find it to imagine the path ahead for a patient? Can you imagine multiple pathways and how they might unfold differently?
- How comfortable are you with the 'chronic unease' of constantly scanning for threats to patient recovery? Does this provoke anxiety or a sense of control for you?

Reading the Waves

You have to have a moderately high emotional IQ. I think if you are unable to read the room you will struggle. You have to be able to see the struggle of others; you have to be able to see the fear in others; you have to be able to see the anguish in others. Whether it's the family, or the patient, or your peers, or your

colleagues or the nurses. If you don't see that, if you can't sense that, you'll miss a lot of opportunities to be a leader, and to be effective.

- How easy do you find it to recognise the emotional needs of others?
- If you find it hard to recognise the emotional needs of others, what strategies have you developed to deal with this?
- Think of an example where you might have 'read the room' better. What was it that made it that situation more challenging?
- Can you think of situations where you witnessed strong emotions in others? How did it make you feel and how did it impact your care?
- While empathy is being able to 'put yourself in the place of others', compassion is using that understanding to guide your actions. Can you think of an example where you were able to use your emotional understanding to positively influence care?
- What strategies do you use to ensure you remain emotionally connected to others but don't become overwhelmed by their emotions? Can you think of examples where this has been more difficult?

Gliding Over the Water

I try to make a point of being very consistent… I try and be the same if things are going well or if they're not going well. I think if there's something, if there is an acute event or a complication going on, I think if you show that you are tempered, it keeps other people calm. If you start getting frazzled and being short and rude, and dropping things, I think that it's very counter-productive. So even if I'm stressed inwardly, I'd deliberately try and outwardly appear to be docile.

- We have previously presented the analogy of the intensivist as a duck, seemingly gliding over water while furiously paddling below the surface. Do you recognise 'ducks' within your ICU, appearing calm and in control despite the demands of the situation?
- What advantages does this approach have for the team in an ICU environment?
- Are there any disadvantages to being a 'duck' or having one as your leader?
- How easy do you find it regulate your own emotions in the moment? What makes this easier or more difficult for you?
- Can you think of a time where you became overtly frustrated or angry in your clinical work? What was the situation and what made it so challenging? What were the impacts on you and the team?
- Do you think the ability to regulate emotions is something intrinsic to an individual, or is it something you develop over time? How might you develop this ability in your practice?

What Kind of Swimmer Are You?

I'm much more introspective, like most intensivists are… Extroverted people tend to work out things in space, okay, with other people. Introverts try and make sense of it, and then only present it to the space when they feel safe and have processed it and packaged it to some extent.

I'm on the introverted side, but I don't have trouble getting along with most people… But… when you are dealing with a frustrated short-tempered surgeon, and I'm trying to navigate… I can do it; it just makes me uncomfortable.

- In intensive care medicine, there is a need to be thoughtful about the best care for patients, yet in certain situations there is a need for immediate action. How do you recognise which approach is needed? Do you find it easy to switch between approaches?
- How easy is it for you to recognise the 'bigger picture' of what is going on for a patient? How has this changed over time?
- Do you tend to work through issues by talking about them, or do you process them internally? What do you see as the advantages and disadvantages of each approach?
- If you tend to process issues internally, how do you make sure the wider team understands the situation and rationale for the plan?
- How do you find working as part of a team? Are you energised by it, or do you find it tiring?
- How do you recharge when you are feeling drained? Do you seek company, or do you take some time away from others?
- When are you most comfortable working as part of a team? What makes it more challenging?

Diving In

Lack of assertiveness can be a problem…. Like somebody who is more experienced says "I think we should do this", and you think maybe that's not quite right but [You think] you've been doing this for 25 years so probably you know where things are headed better than I do". And then, two hours later, you wished you had had voiced your opinion. So that does happen….

I have become more assertive… I'm a bit more, umm, not someone who you can ignore and disrespect… "This is my space, my unit, I'm looking after it, these are my patients, and you're communicating with me, and we are going to talk about this".

- One of the challenges in ICU is how to discuss complex issues, valuing different viewpoints yet avoiding disrespect. Can you identify a past case where disagreement in the team led to a richer understanding of the situation? What made that discussion work?

- How does it make you feel when there is disagreement or conflict?
- Reflect on a situation where you were not confident in asserting yourself. What did you learn?
- How does it feel to hold a different opinion from other people?
- What makes it easier or harder for you to share your views with others?
- How do you feel when your views are dismissed by others? What about when you 'win' an argument? How does it change your relationship with those involved?
- You may not be a naturally assertive person, but sometimes assertion is needed to advocate for patient care. What approaches have you seen that support being assertive without being confrontational?

A Magnificent Work in Progress

You have to recognise that if you admit you're imperfect, it's not like an imposter syndrome where you will be found out or have failed. Everybody who gets here was at the top of the class at some point in their schooling. No 'D' students got to this point. So yes, you have to ask for help (emotionally), but the soil has to be fertile and tilled, and that only comes from inside… if you're not in a place to hear that, you are not going to be receptive.

- Why did you study medicine? Is it what you thought it would be?
- How did you end up choosing intensive care medicine?
- Can you recognise your own achievements in getting to this place in your career? What has helped you to succeed so far? Who encouraged you along the way?
- Have you ever felt like an imposter in your career as a doctor? What triggered that feeling?
- What are you most interested in learning about now? Has this changed from past interests?
- How do you know what you need to work on? Whose opinions do you seek out?
- How do you feel about intensivists who are open about their fallibility and imperfections? Does it affect the way you feel about them positively or negatively?

The Unknowable Ocean of Knowledge

(You think) … that you can do everything; you should know everything; Now, I realise I don't know everything, and I probably never will know everything, but I can always know more today than I did the day before; and I can keep working on it; and it's a process; and I don't control everything.

(You need) a pretty healthy appreciation that you don't know everything, and that you're going to be wrong some of the time. Because you are definitely in a specialty, we are constantly seeking advice and expertise from other specialties or trying to pull together the expertise of multiple teams.

- The breadth of knowledge relevant to ICU means that it is essentially unknowable by a single person. Although everyone aspires to know more, how comfortable are you that you will never know everything?
- How does it feel to ask for help from others? What makes it easier or harder for you?
- Have you experienced a situation where a senior doctor asked for help in providing options in an acute setting? How did it make you feel?
- Is it something you have done and if so, how did it make you feel? Did you experience repercussions in the moment or later from the people who were involved in that experience with you?
- If you have never asked for help like this, consider why? Is it because you have not needed help, or were you worried about how it would change people's perception of you?
- We work as part of multiple teams, bringing our combined expertise to bear on the complex problems of the critically unwell. How does it feel to be dependent on others to deliver the best care possible? Does it affect your perception of your role in the team?

In Shifting Waters

Getting to a point of accepting that uncertainty is part of what we do. You can never be sure. It's part of something that I think the trainees have to learn. A lot of them struggle with not being 100% sure. You've got to be okay with, "There is some uncertainty here" you know? And as long as you have a plan to deal with Outcome A, versus Outcome B, and you know what you are going to do, most of the time it's okay. It was stressful for me in the beginning … not always being sure … but now I realise that that's part of it.

- Intensive care involves time-critical decision-making, often in the face of ambiguous and uncertain problems. The intensivist's job can be seen as 'judgment in the face of uncertainty', meaning decisions must be made even when the correct choice isn't clear. How has your training prepared you for dealing with uncertainty?
- How will you navigate and communicate uncertainty to patients, their families, and members of the healthcare team? What strategies have you used or observed?
- A common saying in ICU is "the answer to every question is: it depends", highlighting how contextual factors constantly shape our decisions. How have you experienced this in your career? Has it changed over time?

- Uncertainty can be challenging to our professional identity. We mistake the uncertainty of a situation for some inadequacy in ourselves. Have you experienced this in your career? If so, how did it affect you?
- Given the inherent uncertainty, things will sometimes not go as expected. What strategies do you have to be 'safely wrong'?

Confidently Cautious

If you become a senior attending and you are so arrogant to think that the second you show up, you'll figure it out… you're going to be a dangerous doctor. Kids can humble you in a second… But I have gotten enough experience to be mature enough to know that even after my best efforts, the child could die. So, you have to be careful that you don't come in and stick your chest out and say everything is going to be good, because that just means you don't know what you're doing. But at the same time, you also… I can instinctively put in lines and do CPR and callout meds so efficiently (clicks fingers), that if I just go into motion, I'm going to feel like I'm giving this patient the best opportunity to pull through.

- What do you see as the difference between confidence and arrogance?
- Can you recall being in a team where the leader seemed anxious and uncertain? What was it like being in that team? How did it impact the team performance?
- Can you recall being in a team where the leader didn't listen to others or was dismissive of different ideas? What was it like being in that team? How did it affect the team performance?
- How do you balance being confident in your abilities yet open to being wrong? Do you think acknowledging your fallibility undermines your role as the team leader?

Testing the Waters

Be sceptical of both others and what they say to you, not in a disrespectful way but to question what they say, but the most important person to be sceptical of, is yourself. Because you have a bigger blind spot than you can possibly know and so be sceptical of what you think and always be prepared to think that although that's the way you see it and you're probably right, but what if, that's not quite the way things are?

- Given the uncertain and ambiguous nature of the work we do, we often base our decisions on incomplete information and partial understanding of the situation. Our assumptions about a case can then trap us into seeing the world in a certain way, even as things change. Have you experienced or observed a situation like this? How did it progress and what triggered a change in understanding?

- Have you experienced a situation you were certain about something, only to find out later you were mistaken? How did that make you feel? How about when you saw someone else do the same thing?
- Scepticism of others can sometimes come across as arrogance. How do you avoid this trap?
- In your experience, what helps you feel comfortable to raise issues with others, such as mistaken assumptions or missing information?
- What strategies do you have to enable the team to help you see your blind spots? How do you create a shared belief within the team that you their help is wanted?

In Stormy Seas

For me, it never happens in the moment. Like a patient died and… in the moment that something is happening, I am able to separate. I need to manage the situation and carry through… And it's usually afterwards when I'm processing and thinking about the loss that was experienced by someone….

Yes so, I'm a "crier"! I need my time and space to do that.

- There are significant impacts that come from caring for those who are critically ill. We are routinely exposed to some of the most emotionally challenging times in people's lives. This can affect us all, at different times and in different ways. What emotional impacts have you experienced in relation to work? How do you deal with these?
- How safe do you feel to express your emotions with others?
- Who are the people you seek out to help you process your emotions?
- Do these emotional impacts effect your life outside of work? In what way?
- How does it feel to show your emotions with families, such as crying when dealing with a grieving family?
- Do you often express sadness by crying? If so, reflect on what the act of crying does for you.
- If you are not a crier, how do you feel about people who do? Is it a strength, a weakness, or something else entirely?
- Have you ever experienced feelings of inadequacy or even guilt in relation to patient care? What was it about the situation that made you feel that way? How did you work through that?

Conclusion

It is clear from the examples above that an intensive care career has many aspects that are challenging to our sense of self. The dynamic, uncertain, and high-stakes decisions that are required by the job can undermine our sense of mastery. Likewise, the work creates significant emotional demands, which require us to regulate ourselves while supporting others. There is a risk that we mistake these challenges as reflecting personal shortcomings, rather than understanding them as an intrinsic part of the work we do.

While these issues are constant, the way we navigate them will vary between individual intensivists. The hope is that by exploring the questions above, we can begin to understand ourselves better. We see how our past experiences and perspectives shape our strokes as we swim in the challenging and turbulent waters of intensive care.

Chapter 7
Floating, Treading Water, and Swimming: Contemplating Your Role

Peter Vernon van Heerden (iD)

Life's roughest storms prove the strength of our anchors
—*Unknown*

As medical experts in intensive care, or *intensivists*, we have a multi-faceted role every time we step into our workplaces. Sometimes we are floating, waiting to see what might evolve; sometimes we are treading water, biding our time to see if our approach is working; sometimes we are actively swimming—against the tide or with it—to save us from sinking. Often our role is clearly defined, but many times we must meet several requirements at the same time. The so-called CanMEDS criteria (1) of what a medical expert is, as promulgated by the Royal College of Physicians and Surgeons of Canada, best encapsulates the roles we have to fulfil in order to be excellent medical experts/intensivists. The domains defined by these criteria are professional, communicator, collaborator, leader, health advocate and scholar. Exploring some of the quotations below will further clarify the intensivist's role in each situation regarding the components of what a medical expert is.

Extending the Capacity of Medical Support

Another physician will have a patient that they are struggling with on the ward, and the team is uncomfortable, and the nurses are uncomfortable, then we get involved from the ICU. We walk in the room and declare, "Umm, all this patient needs is some oxygen, 2mg/kg of Lasix, and to be suctioned, like, what's wrong with you people"? So, you have to know that about yourself. You have to recognise that the (the other team) is at the limit of their capacity, whereas you

P. V. van Heerden (✉)
Department of Anesthesiology, Critical Care and Pain Medicine, Hadassah University Medical Center, Jerusalem, Israel

© The Author(s), under exclusive license to Springer Nature   53
Switzerland AG 2025
D. Dennis et al. (eds.), *Contemplating the Role of an Intensive Care Doctor*,
https://doi.org/10.1007/978-3-031-92766-9_7

are at the bottom of your capacity. So, then you have to be non-judgemental and welcome. "We are happy to have this patient; I can see this patient is struggling…" You bring them in openly. But some of my colleagues can't do that. There's like, "Here's what you do; I've told you what to do; I've given you five instructions, what's wrong with you? Why didn't you carry out my directives…"? You have to recognise that that's how you are perceived. Now I don't practice that way intentionally, but perhaps I am an outlier. Many of my colleagues, that's exactly what happens. And you'll hear other physicians complain "Oh my gosh, I hate when the ICU physicians come; they are so unimpressed; they give me all these orders and it doesn't help me manage the patient". So, you have to understand what to you is "no big deal", is a total crisis to everyone else.

- When a patient is clinically deteriorating, there are often heightened tensions in the moment. Do you recognise the scenario described—perhaps you needed to call for help from the ward as a junior doctor; perhaps you have attended such a call as an intensivist? Think about that episode. No matter your role, how do you think you were perceived by those around you?
- What did you learn from that experience?
- How did it change you?
- How do you want to be perceived by the team in your role now? As a rescuer/retriever?
- As rescuer/retriever, do you check in with the referring doctors after an event? If you do, what does that look like; if you don't, could or should you?
- As the attending intensivist, how did you think your communication went with the referring team? Did you support them, or did you dismiss them?
- Did you interact with all the members of the referring team to offer encouragement and comfort in what they had already done?
- In such a scenario, how would you endeavour to interact with the patient and their family?
- After an interaction such as described, what feelings would you have as you left the scene—satisfaction at having helped the team and the patient; impatience to get back to the 'real work'; or irritation at having to deal with a 'bunch of clueless people?'
- Consider each of your roles as a leader (as the person to whom everyone in this situation is looking up to for guidance), a professional, a health advocate, and a collaborator in this scenario. Would you fulfil all these roles in the situation described?

Accepting Different Acuity Thresholds

I've had situations where I get a phone call, particularly from an outlying facility – and I understand; I see critically ill children for a living, and I see them every day that I am on clinical service, and so what I deem to be "on death's doorstep" and what a community pediatrician or emergency physician in a

community hospital that sees a dozen critically ill kids in a year – I picked that number out of the sky – is very different. They may say, "This kid looks terrible", and by the time they get to me, they are happy and laughing and really don't need to be in the ICU; but for them, it's sick.

- Different facilities have different thresholds of acuity based on their resources and experience. Imagine yourself working in a place where you had inadequate equipment to manage a deteriorating patient, despite having the skillset to do so. How do you feel?
- Now imagine yourself receiving this patient at your well-equipped facility. As described, on arrival the patient looks relatively stable and 'well'. You are experiencing significant capacity demands in your unit, you elect to safely transfer the patient to the general ward. Do you check in with the referring doctors? If you do, what approach do you take; if you don't, could or should you?
- How well do you communicate with the referring doctor to try and ascertain the real reason for transfer of the patient—is it because they are nervous, because they lack experience in dealing with the condition, or because of inadequate resources etc.?
- Would you consider yourself judgemental in this type of situation—and perhaps reach judgement without knowing "the full story"?
- What would your approach be to the parents of the patient if you did decide to send the patient to a general ward and not the ICU in your establishment? How would you explain the 'needless' transfer of the patient?
- Consider your roles as a professional and a collaborator (to the referring physician) and how you would demonstrate this to the parents of the child who was referred.

Saving the Day

I certainly don't think that we are the smartest; but watching a seasoned intensivist instinctively save a person's life is pretty cool; just the CPR; the airway; the breathing; the coordination of all of that. And I'm pretty good at it now because I've done it for so long; it's like, that's my skill set, and I think it can be perceived as… You know, I'll go down to the ER and there will be a grey child who is very close to death, and you just go into this rhythm, and you resuscitate aggressively, and regardless of the outcome, there's sort of a big sigh of relief when the intensivist comes down. Because you've got the most likely person that's going to help. I think throughout the hospital, the feeling is that the ICU attending is there… Yeah… A sigh of relief, that they're there….

- This high level of expectation is probably entirely reasonable, as the intensivist may have the best chance of retrieving the situation. Take a moment to consider how the expectation might also be a significant stressor for the intensivist. How do you think you might deal with those expectations?

- Would this change if you were unable to successfully retrieve a situation, and the patient died?
- In some circumstances, do you think that this high level of expectation might facilitate a perception of rescuer/retriever arrogance on the part of the referrer?
- Do you check in with the referring doctors after an event? If you do, how do you achieve that; if you don't, could or should you?
- One of the most important roles to fill in this situation is that of leader. How well do you think you take on this role, as the person most skilled to undertake the clinical tasks needed?
- What is the role of communication whilst acting as the leader?
- With leadership comes responsibility. Arriving at a scene of high stress, with very little prior knowledge and not having met the patient/the parents before, how do you cope with taking charge of the situation?
- If the outcome is not good, do you take responsibility for the outcome even though you may have been the last person on the scene?

Prevention

Everything you do is a potential error, waiting to happen, isn't it? If you do it poorly, and so, that's part of supervision and leading. A lot of the things you do to pre-empt any mistakes that might happen, because if you just let everything run its course I think a lot more mistakes would happen, and that's why you are there, in charge. And so a lot of the communication, the way you set things up as to what's going to happen next… I talk through a lot about what's going to happen, why are we doing this, what are we going to do and I guess that is the whole point, is to pre-empt errors.

- It is often easier to presume that the intensivist occupies the role of 'protector' rather than 'protagonist' in the patient journey through acuity, but in the high-stakes area of intensive care medicine, the sheer number of invasive high-risk procedures performed potentiates error. Have you considered your role in error prevention within the intensive care environment itself?
- What pragmatic steps do you take every day to minimise the number of mistakes you make?
- What pragmatic steps do you take every day to minimise the number of mistakes your team makes?
- Clearly leadership, professionalism and communication are the major roles required as an intensivist to mitigate mistakes. How do you fit into each of these roles?
- Acting as an example is very important in setting the tone in an ICU—'do as I say and as I do' rather than 'do as I say and don't worry how I do it'. Can you think of other examples where leading by example is effective, such as hand hygiene, sticking to protocol during invasive procedures?

- In the ICU we work as a team, and making sure the whole team knows what the current therapeutic goals are is very important. What is the role of communication in the team setting?
- Errors are inevitable in a busy ICU. How do you cope when you make a serious, life-threatening error? What strategies do you employ that allow you to come back to work the next day?

Pushing the Envelope

I think from a medical perspective you have to teach people not to be risk adverse. Because stasis is death. Every day in the ICU is bad; every day… we are the enemy, right? The car accident was the car accident; the cardiac surgery was the cardiac surgery; the pneumonia was the pneumonia. Everything that happens after that we are responsible for. So the goal is not to be stable, the goal is to be constantly pushing the envelope. What does this patient not need today? What can we get away with removing or stopping? And don't just assume that they can't, prove it. And if you don't constantly push that, you lose patients, you kill people. Because you add days to the ICU care; you add days on the ventilator; you add days to that toxic medicine; you add days to central IV access. So you have to have risk tolerance, you have to not be afraid to be wrong 10 or 15 % of the time. If you're waiting for that certainty, you're killing patients. You have to learn that.

- Sometimes 'pushing the envelope' is viewed by the wider healthcare team as being unsafe, putting patients at higher risk, rather than protective. An early extubation, for example, does it prevent a ventilator acquired pneumonia but cause an aspiration pneumonia? A shared understanding of the team that the intensive care environment is a risk is important to build and convey. How do you do this?
- In a setting of prognostic uncertainty, will the patient maintain their airway after extubation, or will they not?—how do you convey to your team that your decisions are carefully considered?
- How do you cope with having your decisions questioned by your team?
- How do you manage your team when your hunches are wrong?
- When working in a team, how do you prevent the medical decisions being made based on intuition not becoming outlandish or 'experimental'?
- How important is the role of scholar when making medical decisions to advance the progress of a patient in the ICU, i.e. knowing all the medical options available?
- Another important role of the intensivist in the ICU therapeutic team is to be a health advocate. How so you balance this role regarding the patient in front of you, with the needs of all the patients in the ICU, the hospital and society as a whole?

- Do you think asking the following question/s at the end of each case presentation during a ward round is reasonable and useful? 'Why is this patient still on a ventilator'? 'Why is the patient on vasopressors'? 'Why is the patient in the ICU'?

Transitioning to Palliative Care

I think you have to recognise that death and life are part of the same journey. And your mission in life cannot be to extinguish one and welcome the other. You have to find balance and practice towards both goals. Every excellent intensivist in my opinion is also an outstanding palliative care physician, and if they are separate in your mind, I mean providing good ICU care and being a palliative care doctor, you've missed the entire point. Because as I tell all my trainees, for how many years have there been healers, physicians? 3000, 4000, more? How many of those years could they do anything? Maybe 125? So, what did they do for the other 2944 years? They held your hand. They were... your guide. So, to me, that role of the physician as a "healer" is to recognise when it's my job to guide and hold your hand and when it's my job to put a breathing tube into you and give you everything I have in the hospital. And if you can't recognise that both roles are yours, then I think you're missing a huge component of what it means to be an intensivist. You are the person who can guide that family towards living or toward death. A death with dignity is a gift; a resuscitation leading to ongoing life is a gift. To do them both well is our job. So, you need to be able to recognise when to mode switch. But it's a continuum. It's not like A or B. It's a continuum of understanding.

- Some intensive care doctors see palliative care as a core role of their profession. Is it something you have considered?
- What skills and attributes do you think you need to have to be able to explore a patient's wishes?
- Do you think you possess these? What could you work on to be more confident in having these conversations?
- Have you ever needed to deliver bad news to a patient? If so, how did it go? If not, have you ever practised that scenario out aloud?
- What skills and attributes do you think you need to have to do this well? Do you think you possess these? What could you work on to be more confident in having these conversations?
- How would you navigate a conversation where a patient and their family have conflicting wishes?
- Making the mental switch to move from intensive care to palliative care is not one that all intensivists can easily make—can you identify some of the factors that might prevent this mental switch?
- How do you think you balance the instinct to rescue with empathy for the dying patient?

- Do you think it's always right to 'do everything' for every patient in the ICU? If so, what does 'everything' mean, given that ECMO is now a common modality?
- Who do you consult with when considering palliation?
- Does palliative care always mean end-of-life care to you, or does it have a broader meaning, for example, providing symptom control?
- How do you deal with conflicts within the team or between the ICU team and the 'home' team (e.g. surgeons) about the appropriateness or otherwise of palliation? Who has the final say about the direction of treatment?
- As a 'rational' medical expert, do you rely on spiritual guidance when making end-of-life decisions? If so, does this help and support you?
- When considering palliation, all the following roles of the medical expert are required—professional, communicator, health advocate, leader, scholar and collaborator. How would you fulfil each role in making the decision to move from intensive care to palliative care?

Privilege

I think one of the great privileges of medicine for me has been… I think it's made me more humble and empathetic than I would have been had I been in a different profession… It's a privilege to be invited to be part of another person's narrative during a very stark time. And that has informed my appreciation for my own experiences in my own life.

- Have you arrived at a place in your career where you can genuinely relate to this notion of 'privilege' that so many intensivists expressed?
- For some intensivists, 'privilege' mitigates the burden of the job. For others, the importance of these moments becomes a burden, as it adds to their performance anxiety—'I must do this well, because it's such a privilege to be undertaking this role with the family'. Which viewpoint do you have, and does it hinder or enhance your ability to convey care to a patient and their family during these times?
- How do you relate this notion of privilege back to your own life?
- Together with privilege comes great responsibility. We are dealing with patients at their most vulnerable, and a word or a gesture out of place can have a great and lasting effect on the patient and their family. How do you deal with this responsibility on a daily basis, given that you are 'only human' and also have 'off' days?
- It's easy to be distracted by the technical aspects of work in the ICU—doses of powerful medications, ventilator settings and placing lines—but as an intensivist, how do you act as an example of empathic care of very sick patients?
- How do you conduct a conversation with the family of a critically ill patient to convey both the medical facts and situation together with showing empathy? Where and when do such conversations take place?

- How do you judge your level of empathy—by what you think or by what others say about you?
- How often do staff and family compliment you on your kind treatment of patients and their families?

Showing Emotion in the Moment

I personally don't cry a lot in any part of my life. Not out of coldness. Like sometimes I wish I could cry but... Some people can cry all the time at anything... And it's a release... I don't know if it just wasn't modelled for me a lot... While I don't cry, it's not out of complete stoicism, is out of, just who I am.

I get teary-eyed in... mostly in meetings; mostly in discussions, rather than being at the bedside... and I think it's good. I think there is a very big human to human thing... that if you come across as a robot, they will have the memory of some cyborg taking care of their kid... And then I think they definitely appreciate and are soothed by the compassion that a tear shows.

I sometimes (cry), yeah – more when we are nearing the end of life and I can see that our efforts are not going to be successful, and we are talking through with families about how it's going to be, and that's sad... I don't know if it's healing. And I've actually felt guilty for doing that. And forcing parents to in a way, care for me. For them to see me suffering with them I think might be an emotional burden that I don't want to burden them even further. On the other side, I wonder if parents find some feeling of healing from knowing that as a provider....

- As the quotes suggest, some people cry easily, and some don't. Where are you on that continuum broadly in your life?
- Is that different or much the same in your workplace?
- Would you allow yourself to cry with the patient and their family?
- Do you think it serves a purpose for the family?
- Do you think it serves a purpose for you?
- How do you feel when you see another member of your team shed a tear?
- Some people believe that exhibiting emotion demonstrates empathy. How effective do you think showing emotion is as a communication tool?
- Do you think crying is somewhat selfish in that now the patient and their family might think they need to comfort you? Or could it be that they now see that you are also moved by their situation and 'stand with them'?
- Besides crying, what other non-verbal cues could be used to convey empathy for suffering patients and families?
- How important is non-verbal communication as a tool when dealing with patients and families?

Regulating the Room

I think that if I'm in room of people that are… Or at least it appears to me they're not able to regulate… Like they're having difficulty with regulating the expanse of emotions that are happening, I try to maintain as regulated a state as I can to try to help provide the best support that I can. But I do think there are times when it's… And maybe I'm reading it wrong, that it's helpful… But it may be helpful for a family to see that you are moved by the experience that they are having… I try not to add when I clearly see that there is a room that seems uncontrolled, people are overly emotional, but I also think that sometimes at least it appears that your emotional response lets the family know that you are there with them, and that you understand their experience. Even if you don't know what it is, that you are with them in the moment….

- In some overly emotional circumstances, a high level of emotional intelligence is required to be able to 'read the room' and de-escalate the situation appropriately. What does 'reading the room' mean to you?
- Have you been in a setting where the room was not regulated and emotions were high?
- If you have, what controlled the environment and who led this? What did you learn from this in terms of what to do and what not to do?
- If you have not, can you think of what devices you might employ to contain the emotion and regulate the atmosphere?
- How would you deal with verbal abuse directed at you or other staff in the ICU. For example, 'You are all murderers. He was fine when he came in and now he's dead – and you did this'!
- How would you deal with physical violence against you or other staff in the ICU?
- Is there ever a situation where 'discretion is the better part of valour' and leaving the scene is appropriate, to come back later and try and talk rationally?
- What is your approach to situations such as described above, but were there might be a language or cultural barrier?
- How do you modify your approach if substances like drugs or alcohol are involved in influencing the behaviour in the room?
- If appropriate body language and tone of voice are not calming the situation in the room, is it justified to raise your voice and take a dominant or commanding tone?
- Do you think all situations as described can be dealt with rationally?

Guiding the Room; Guiding the Family

I think you have to be able to span the spectrum of allowing your genuine self to be in the room, to allowing the room itself to guide your actions. And you're also their guide, right? You're creating this scenario; you're creating the

desired outcome. **No matter how you want to call it, you can't be a good intensivist if you don't understand the timing and the role and heavy handedness and the paternalism at play. Now I'm not suggesting that all medical care is one-sided, I'm suggesting that these people have never been in this position before. To this family the death of a child is new to them. You have been in that scenario 20 or 30 or 40 or 100 times. You cannot absolve yourself of the responsibility of (being) their guide. Which means you have to have a destination, and that means that in some way or another, you have to guide them even as you read them. You could argue that that is inherently paternalistic. If you go into every encounter with no agenda, and no direction, and you are just like a passive guide for which the family is going to take you on, you are going to struggle, I tell you right now. You absolutely have to learn when and how that journey needs to be shaped, and not too much, and not too little, and it takes a lot of practice.**

- This quote elegantly described the notion of the intensivist as an expert guide towards death. Have you ever considered one of your roles to be this?
- If you are more junior in your role, it may be tricky for you to consider. How might you prepare yourself for this?
- What responsibility does the role convey to you?
- You may have heard stories from your colleagues around their good and not so good experiences in doing this well. What have you learned?
- Is this part of the job that you consider is (or will be) difficult or fulfilling? Why?
- In dealing with this type of conversation, do you see yourself as 'the captain of the ship' or more as 'the pilot' guiding the ship through rough seas? Which role do you think would be more effective?
- Dealing with difficult conversations effectively is an acquired skill. What, in your opinion, is the role of mentorship in acquiring these skills? Who did you learn from, and if you are junior, who do you hope to learn from?
- What would you consider a satisfactory outcome to such a conversation—for you and for the family?
- If a difficult conversation does not go satisfactorily, what do you do? For example, would you terminate the conversation and suggest a conversation at another time; call for help; and display your own emotion?
- How do you decompress after a difficult family conversation in a way that allows you to continue working and come back for another such conversation on another day?
- Do you readily take on difficult conversations as part of your role, or do you try and avoid them? Why?
- Are you aware of the words or actions in others that might trigger your fight, flight and anger responses to control these emotions?
- How do you avoid appearing defensive when confronted by aggressive relatives?
- Is it ever justified to lie during a family discussion to avoid a difficult topic, even if it's a 'white' lie?

- How do you cope if you feel that there is no trust and that the family is suspicious of everything you and the staff say or do, implying that you have something to hide?
- Is 'open disclosure' of any accidents or incidents that might have led to a poor outcome always the best policy?

Not Having All the Answers

Oftentimes you don't have the answers to everything, and parents want answers. And sometimes even just telling them "I don't know". We don't know the diagnosis for instance; there are some kids where we've done a million-dollar work up and we are still struggling to come up with a unifying diagnosis to put everything together. Or sometimes, I don't know exactly what we should do next. You know I'm gonna talk to some colleagues or just saying, "I don't know" I think, for instance, and I find that most families actually receive that well. I think most families see that as… I've hardly seen anybody who gets upset when you say, "You don't know". I think they appreciate that you are being open and honest and are willing to saying that you don't know: "I'll be darned, we haven't seen this before, I don't know".

- Intensivists train extensively to prepare for the conditions that present and the treatment options they can offer, but no one can know everything! How does the quotation above resonate with you? Is it easy for you to be fallible with your patients and their families?
- Consider the downside of offering this transparency? How might you manage these sequelae?
- Now consider the upside. What positives might come of you being open and honest and willing to admit that 'you don't know'?
- The medical expert roles involved in this scenario include 'scholar', knowing as much as possible, but not possibly knowing everything; 'leader', even if everything is not known, then at least setting the direction to find out; 'collaborator', looking for advice wherever necessary; and 'communicator', keeping everyone on the team and in the patient's family informed. Have you considered how you would undertake each of these roles in this situation?
- Does being fallible make us any less professional?
- Is obfuscation—'fake it until you make it'—ever justified in this situation? Why?

Responsibility

I am the responsible entity. That's not really me personally, but the position that I hold is the responsible entity. I kinda think that the family probably think that to. I am the face of the health system that is now talking to them. I am the health system as far as they're concerned, right? And health system has done this, so I don't think I am personally responsible. Oftentimes they will say that. I usually don't feel personally responsible if events have occurred beyond my ability to control. But I suppose I am hierarchically or institutionally responsible because I am sitting in the chair that is the health system and they are sitting in a chair that is the family.

I think there is a legal view, and I guess there is a moral view, and I guess there is a professional view. I think the legal view would be that the person in charge of the ICU at the time has some ultimate responsibility for what's going on. I think the moral view is that that person may not even know something is happening, and there would be other actors involved who are directly potentially responsible for contacting the person or not contacting the person, so it is difficult to allocate responsibility to a person who didn't know anything was actually happening. And so those are different. And I think there is the clinical professional view, that says that it is the interaction between the person responsible and the person at the coalface in the 24-hour cycle that is responsible for it. So, one says, "You are the person responsible", it's like the Westminster system - you're the Prime Minister, down you go. The other one says, "Look, I didn't even know this was happening, how can I be responsible"? "Morally, how can I be responsible? These guys are doing all this stuff, and I didn't even know"? And the third one says, "Well, you should have known, and the fact that you didn't know is your responsibility as well as their responsibility, because they should have told you. But you should have created a culture where they should have told you. And the fact that they didn't tell you, is your responsibility as well as theirs".

- There are moral and ethical arguments around 'responsibility' in the intensive care, but for both patients and their families, as a lead doctor, you are likely the face of the healthcare system. As a result, many intensivists view that the accountability and responsibility of all care ultimately rest with them. Do you share that opinion?
- How do you reconcile that the mistakes of others may lie with you as the lead intensivist?
- As the quotation states, there are several aspects to responsibility, personal, moral, institutional and legal. Can you think of situations where each type of responsibility has fallen on you?
- Do you feel that you have institutional backup (support from your administration) for your taking responsibility for the institution?

- Do each of personal, moral, institutional and legal responsibility carry the same weight with you? Which type of responsibility affects you most?
- Discuss the importance of communication and documentation when dealing with responsibility for an adverse event.
- When is it necessary and/or permissible to share the responsibility with others, for example, the hospital legal or risk management team or malpractice insurers?
- Is the head of the intensive care department the responsible 'adult' for all activities in the department? Or is he/she only the face/spokesperson for all events in the ICU?
- How important is it to debrief as a team after an adverse event?
- Once an adverse event has been discussed in an open forum such as a morbidity and mortality (M&M) meeting, is it also reasonable to ascribe personal responsibility for the outcome to an individual in the meeting (once it becomes clear who was indeed responsible)? How will such an approach affect participation in M&M meetings?

Conclusion

This chapter has been about the intensivist contemplating their role in the workplace. The quotations and the related questions strive to illustrate that intensivists are not and cannot be black and white or unimodal. Each of us as healthcare providers is required to inhabit several roles and personas in our daily work, depending on the situation we find ourselves in. As discussed in Chap. 6, it takes a degree of self-awareness to know what our strengths are and which of the personas we best inhabit, as related to our personalities and abilities. As an extension, some may find certain roles easier than others, and although this may be true, intensivists need to perform all the roles as outlined in this chapter—from the leader to the scholar to the communicator. Knowing that we are part of a therapeutic team and that we can also rely on those around us to support us in the roles we may not feel so accomplished at is important.

Reference

1. https://canmeds.royalcollege.ca/guide. Accessed on 1st July 2024.

Chapter 8
The Stormy Sea: Contemplating the Place

Aaron Calhoun ⬤

> *Rough seas make stronger sailors. Tough times build greater people.*
>
> –Robin Sharma

Like a stormy sea, the ICU environment is both complex and challenging, and learning the skills required to successfully navigate it can take decades. Most practitioners choose this environment deliberately, in many cases due to the exciting, cognitively rich nature of the medicine, as well as the opportunity to make an immediate difference in the life of their patients. Over time, however, this acuity can also prove emotionally taxing and potentially result in burnout.

The following quotes illustrate key components of this environment, such as the level of acuity, emotional intensity of the care needed and frequent uncertainty regarding the patient's ultimate outcome, as seen through the eyes of current practitioners. Some of these are situations that you may have encountered in your own practice so far, and some may be novel. Sailors and fishermen are drawn to seas and accept the possibility of peril; they may lose their direction, encounter storms or even suffer damage to their vessels. They set out knowing that there is also beauty and bounty in those waters. The intensivist similarly launches into the 'ICU' sea and is the captain on the amazing voyage that is this chosen career.

A. Calhoun (✉)
Department of Pediatric and Norton Children's Medical Group, University of Louisville, Louisville, KY, USA
e-mail: aaron.calhoun@louisville.edu

The Acuity of the Environment

I guess that one thing I always find comforting is that I know my patients are sick. It's not like you are a GP (general practitioner) and have someone in front of you with a headache and you're not sure whether it's a headache or a brain tumour. They've been admitted to ICU so they're obviously sick.

- Reflecting on this statement, does knowing the acknowledged acuity of the ICU patient offer you reassurance as the treating doctor or make you more nervous? Why?
- Now, spend some time considering the word 'sick'. What does this word mean in an ICU environment, in an emergency department (ED) environment, in a ward environment and in the community?
- How does this difference in perception translate to the assessment of a 'sick' patient on an outlying ward whose team is requesting transfer to intensive care? Is it easy for you to identify when the ward where they are currently on is ill equipped to manage the acuity, or it is sometimes a grey area left for you to define?
- Reflect on any events you may have experienced where you differed with a ward or ED team on whether a patient merited ICU admission. What factors do you think led to this difference? How were any conflicts resolved?
- How do you navigate any uncertainty you feel, and what are the checks and balances you put in place to ensure that the patient remains safe on a ward if you choose to leave them there?
- How does the knowledge that your patients most likely are suffering from significant, and potentially life-threatening, illness affect your emotional status when preparing for a shift? Do you find it energizing or a source of anxiety?
- How do these emotions impact your immediate family relationships or your relationships with friends?
- What resources have you used in the past to deal with the emotional stress of this environment?
- What resources are available that you might be able to use in the future? Are you actively considering any at present?

Around the Clock Care

…A surgeon is called, and then a different surgeon comes on in the morning; An intensivist is called overnight, and then a different intensivist comes on in the morning. And then a lot of conflict in the morning between none of the people who were actually there, that could speak to it, except for me. (I remember) that being a very unpleasant thing to be a part of. Especially as a junior person where all the decisions were made above me by people who weren't there to… defend the decision-making. And it didn't help anything—none of us learned more by the conflict.

- The nature of the ICU environment is that care continues around the clock, and there is a multitude of personnel from different teams and specialties rotating though to manage and deliver that care. It is therefore no wonder that communication is challenging and multi-layered; handovers are complex; and tensions are often high. With this in mind, and in the context of a deteriorating patient in the middle of the night, how might you anticipate conflict between specialities?
- How might you manage disagreements?
- If you have had such an experience as the one described, what did you learn from it?
- In your experience, has the process of handoff between shifts resulted in important information about medical decisions being lost? If so, how did you respond when you became aware of it?
- Did this loss of information cause any conflict between you and the patient or their family, and between you and other members of the care team?
- Did the experience alter your practice at all?
- How did you deal with the experience emotionally?
- As part of the ICU team, you are required often to work difficult shifts, such as overnights, weekends and holidays throughout your career, and will thus potentially miss events with family and friends for the sake of the patients you care for. Have you considered this reality? Have you had preparatory conversations with your family and friends about this?

Acknowledging the Experience of Others and the Things That Come with That

If you are young, and you say "I don't know what to do", then they (those around you) think that you don't know what to do. If you're older … I can usually get away with it: "I don't know what to do, what do you guys think"? I can say that pretty safely. But a younger person when they say that, then the nurse will come back and say, "Hey, so-and-so doesn't know what they're doing". So, they get caught in the middle. They have to almost pretend they know what to do even though in reality, nobody knows what to do.

And if you are too convinced that you are ready (and) know what the right treatment course is, then you are not actually going to benefit from the different expertise that comes through the unit.

- In a place like ICU, there will always be a spectrum of experience across the providers. Some senior nurses, for example, might have seen more cases of a certain type of pathology than you have seen as a more junior doctor. Have you ever perceived more experienced staff as being judgmental related to your decision-making in the context of your inexperience? How did that make you feel, and how did you respond?

- Pretending to know more than you do is dangerous. Have you ever felt the need to 'fake it until you make it' in the intensive care environment? What did this feel like and how did you keep the patient safe?
- Conversely, it is often difficult to 'feel' confident in new situations, even if you have the objective knowledge and skill to handle it. Have you ever considered how to approach these crises in confidence?
- Listening to the opinions of others is often very useful, and shared decision-making is powerful; however, as a team leader, deferring decision-making completely can be risky for the patient while potentially undermining your own confidence. Can you relate to a situation like this? How might you garner respect while being transparent about your lack of experience?
- Remember, despite your inexperience you may well be choosing the right path. Senior staff with lots of experience can make mistakes too. Consider how you might communicate that your decision was the right one retrospectively to a more senior colleague who had advocated for a different decision in the moment.
- Broadly speaking, how do you deal with over-confident co-workers who regards themselves as more experienced and knowing than you?
- Intensivists can often develop a deep connection to their own thought processes and approaches to the exclusion of those of others. This can often manifest in conflict during transfer of care or sign-out. What techniques might be helpful in overcoming these conflicts?
- Having a humble approach towards the ideas and styles of others can often lead to better care and a more cohesive plan. What preparations can you make to engage in this manner?

Coping with the Continuum of Life

I sat down with her family and was asking them what they wanted, and she said she didn't want an operation, and she wanted to be going to hospice. And the daughter said to me you're the first person that has actually sat down with us in the bedspace and asked us, explained what was going on, and asked us what we wanted… I guess when I first started in ICU I thought of that as a disappointment, or as a thing that was not sort of… I grumbled, but it was not our core business, but now I actually don't mind doing that in that I think that it is probably our role as well, because we probably see from the start to the end a bit better than some of the others, some of the other specialties.

- You might expect to save lives in the ICU, but preparing for death is also important. Consider the role of ICU care within the continuum of life in a palliative care situation—how can you make the ICU a place where patients and their families can emotionally prepare for death?
- Consider the discussion you would have with a patient's family to help them prepare for the death of their loved one within the ICU. What are the key aspects you will cover and clarify?

- Now, consider the impact of the patient's decline on the healthcare team. How might the process affect the nurses, the respiratory therapists and the other clinicians? What support can be provided for them?
- In the ICU, death can occur in several different ways: cardiac death due to an arrest, withdrawal of life sustaining treatment and declaration of brain death. How might these modes of death be perceived as similar by families? How might they be perceived differently? How would you prepare families differently for these experiences?
- An important part of death in the ICU is the prospect of organ donation. The relationship between the intensivist and the organ provider organization can vary greatly, and conflicts can sometimes occur. How might you be able to bridge this gap in your own practice?
- Consider the impact that the above conversations might have on your own sense of well-being. What safeguards can you put in place to enable you to debrief after these difficult events?

Family Members Present

I think that the situation where you have a patient who is coding, or who is very sick, I think that the family presence is important if the family desires it. Now I've had some times where the parents are understandably emotionally upset and crying or screaming, and in that situation I think it can have an adverse effect on the function of the team, so…

It depends on the family. You know if it is a family that you have worked with and they are very suspicious, and they're not trusting, then they need to see that….

For the family. Are they going to have PTSD (post-traumatic stress disorder), having seen that done to their family member? Is that going to be the last memory of their beautiful child'?

- The ICU environment can be a terrifying place to those unfamiliar with it, and the things that take place can be equally frightening to witness. For some families, being present during the resuscitation of their relative is an important part of their acceptance; for others, it may be a confronting trauma that stays with them in a negative way forever. Imagine having a conversation with a family member about their wishes in the event of an emergency procedure for their loved one, in terms of whether they want to be present. What are the key things you would convey?
- What questions do you anticipate them having, and how do you think you might address them?

- Sometimes patients have their own preferences for this. How would you manage a situation where the patient's wishes were different to that of their family?
- Consider the range of emotions the family might display during the event. How do you think the care team might cope with this? How do you think you might cope with this? What measures could you put in place to address the family's emotional needs while you tend to the patient?
- If there is agreement that the family would be present, consider how that decision impacts you and the care you provide.
- Are there any factors that, for you, represent 'no go' criteria for family presence? What are they and why?
- What are the strategies you might consider for your own psychological safety both in preparation for and then during and after the event?

Excessive Emotion from Staff

I think you can't be so emotional that the parents are supporting you. I've seen that happen before; like the nurse is weeping, and the mother is like patting them; and I'm like, "No, no, no". It may not be the nurse's role to comfort the parent, but it's definitely not the parent's role to comfort the nurse.

- Crying at the bedside with the family may be acceptable for some healthcare workers; however, the expression of excessive emotion by a member of the healthcare team can be both burdensome for the family and uncomfortable for co-workers.
- Imagine you are experiencing a situation like the one described in the quotation. Reflect on what you would do in this circumstance in terms of care for the family, care for the team member and care for the team.
- Consider the range of emotions you might experience at the bedside. What do you consider to be personally acceptable and unacceptable means of expressing these?
- Oftentimes your ability to openly express emotion at the bedside is dependent on the type of relationship you have established with the patient and their family. What types of family relationships have you established during your prior training? Consider how this experience might assist you in approaching the above situations.
- Situations that are emotionally difficult for the team, such as the above, have repercussions that extend beyond the event itself. What resources are available at your institution to help with such difficulties?
- Consider how your experience of such events might change over the duration of your career. Do you expect difficult events to have similar impact on you, less, or more?

Heightened Emotion from Family

I did have a gentleman punch a hole in the wall next to my head. That was my first year as a consultant…. I agreed with the sentiment expressed by the fist of this poor grieving husband. I can't recall the details of how I communicated things to him but there was that explosive anger outburst…. getting the right sort of empathy, yes, that's crucial, but I think far more than empathy, is just normalizing and saying it's "It's okay to feel angry, it's okay to feel upset".

I can remember a family, getting very, very angry. Not threatening me physically, but becoming very aggressive to the space around them as a form of grief. And I know that made people feel very threatened and uncomfortable. When they have thought that the patient was coming in for a relatively low risk procedure and they are now critically unwell or have died. I can think of a couple of those incidences where the family are very angry. And I think… we're not well trained always to deal with that anger. And we often don't have spaces set up to allow them to vent, where we can feel safe as well. And when we don't feel safe as a staff group, it's hard to de-escalate that.

- Expression of anger can be a frightening thing to witness in the relatively controlled atmosphere of the ICU. What do you need to consider if you are confronted with the sort of behaviour described in these quotations?
- How do you think the above situation would make you feel? Angry? Threatened? Fearful? How do you think colleagues might react? How might these different internal responses impact your approach?
- What steps would you take to de-escalate the situation?
- Are you aware of the resources available to you within your institution?
- Do you know how to call for help in an escalating situation?
- Have you ever considered the responsibility you might have for the aftercare of co-workers following these traumatic non-clinical episodes? What does this look like for you?
- Consider situations in which you may have witnessed anger of this nature in the past. What was the outcome? Did the family member communicate with you afterwards to apologize or explain? What insights (if any) did this provide on the familial thought process surrounding critical illness?

Balanced Perspective of Outcomes

When nurses start saying, "It's been such a bad stretch… We've had this many deaths…" So we might have had six deaths but we've saved 300 patients! We all remember those really bad things but what about the kid… I remember, it was about a year and a half ago, you know we had a good run on ECMO (extracorporeal membrane oxygenation); a couple of deaths; we just saved a 17 year old's

life and he is at home without a trache, going to prom. Right? Like he's gonna go to college.

- In the context of a disappointing patient outcome, there may be a tendency to catastrophize and lose a balanced perspective. Remembering and even cherishing the good outcomes can be a positive mitigator of emotional distress for providers. How do you think you might facilitate a balanced perspective within your team?
- As you gain experience, it becomes easier for the good outcomes to be seen as 'business as usual', which can give heightened significance to negative outcomes. How might this natural tendency be resisted?
- The type of thoughts and statements above might also be indicators of distress if seen in a colleague. How might you counsel someone experiencing such distress? What resources could you refer them to for assistance?
- Oftentimes difficult stretches such as this can be quite difficult for trainees rotating in the ICU. How might you approach and counsel trainees who are experiencing emotional distress?
- On occasion, ICU clinicians have attended funeral or remembrance services for families with which they have been involved. Others, however, do not do so, seeing this separation as a necessary protective mechanism. Faced with a difficult patient outcome, would you choose to attend memorial services? Why or why not?
- How would you maintain a culture of balance within your unit as a whole?

Balanced Perspective of Failure and Success

"Do you take credit when they get better"? And she said, "No, we give them the medicine and they get better – they're supposed to get better…" And she was like, "So how come you give yourself so much credit for their death"? And I said, "Yeah, you know, we are there to help to the best we can, we're not perfect, nobody is perfect. We don't know what's going to happen tomorrow. If we did, we'd be a whole lot better with this". And so by sort of saying, you need to take as much credit, which is usually not a whole lot for their survival as you do for the death, they need to be equal, and don't beat yourself up for some little thing you did wrong, when you don't give yourself credit for the millions of good things you do.

- Most human beings tend to personalise and ruminate on failure much more than on success. This tendency may be exaggerated in doctors, who are perhaps less familiar with academic failure during the course of their training and who may therefore have a harder time contemplating anything other than success. Do you feel you can celebrate the success of your team in the ICU environment?
- In your own experience, have you ever downplayed a personal or job-related success? If you have, please reflect on the thought process that you believe may have led you to do so.

- If you are having trouble remembering such an occasion, what can you put in place to celebrate a success the next time it happens? How do you think it could impact your workplace culture positively?
  Patients are sick in the ICU, and some of them will go on to live because of what you do. When was the last time you took time to celebrate and remember a patient who lived, and what did you do? Can you reflect on the effect it had on the team you work with and the culture of your workplace?

Relinquishing Control of Outcome

I can do everything absolutely right sometimes and I still have a problem. Or I could be having just an off day all around and nothing is going right but it doesn't make a difference because everything works out. It's just not a predictable process. I guess because of the fact that I can't find an absolute way that you are going to be right all the time, I just sort of say, "Right, well, it was just one of those rolls where I just caught a bad break, and I there's nothing I could do about it".

- Some intensivists conveyed a deep sense of responsibility for the outcome their patients experienced no matter what the circumstances, and so this quotation is important as it recognises that, as a doctor, it is your patient rather than you that is the focus that controls outcome. The ICU is a place where sick people are provided care, and the quality of care imparted at your institution—despite a poor patient outcome—can be a great mitigator of the crushing disappointment of a patient death for both family and provider. Understanding this and being able to share this perspective with your team as the team leader is invaluable. Is this something you have considered?
- Imagine you have been called into a meeting with senior management about setting up a retrieval service, and their concerns centre upon the projected rate of patient survival versus the number of patients who would be offered first class care at your facility with prognosis unknown. What is important to you in terms of the service the intensive care team offers? How would you respond?
- Circumstances often arise when decisions need to be made based on insufficient information, with the potential for higher uncertainty regarding outcome. For some, this can result in significant psychological distress. How might you react to situations such as this?
- Now, consider a hypothetical situation such as this where you believe you made the best decision possible, but the actual outcome was not what was desired. Would you perceive this as stressful? What tools/techniques might be available for you to process this event?
- Individuals often have different baseline tolerances for uncertainty or 'chaos'. For some, this uncertainty is a threat to be mitigated. For others this is a simple fact that must be accepted. How would you classify your own approach? What

communication difficulties might you anticipate between individuals with different approaches to this?

- Consider the cumulative effect of experiences such as the one mentioned in the quote above. How might you expect this to change your attitude towards ICU practice over the span of your career?

Mistakes

I tend to rationalise it by saying, "look, there's complications with any procedure, and if you do enough of them you will have complications from those procedures". And that as long as you can confidently say that you are… that you are current, that you have currency in terms of being able to perform that procedure safely and that you've done… that you got enough experience… that complications will occur, and that is not necessarily anyone's fault it's just a… just a probability.

- The ICU is a place where complex invasive procedures are an everyday practice. It follows therefore that the likelihood of error lies in statistical probability, such that the more you do, the more likely there will be a mistake. On the flipside, it may be true that because the intensivist is likely to repeat these procedures so frequently, they become so adept that the chance of error diminishes. Which school of thinking do you subscribe to?
- Imagine a situation in which you perform a common procedure with which you have significant experience that results in an unforeseen complication. You know that you will need to perform this procedure frequently in the future. What response might you have to this? How would you communicate this with the family? What techniques might assist you in moving past this event so that you can perform your job.
- Consider a situation in which a patient and/or their family files for malpractice due to a complication or error. What resources and/or coping strategies could you employ to assist you in processing the situation?
- A great deal of time and effort is spent within critical care environments to minimize error and promote patient safety. What efforts around these issues are taking place in your current environment? What opportunities exist in which you can become involved? Do you consider it important to be involved in such activities during your future career?
- Consider the relative benefits and risks of checklist-oriented vs critical-thinking-oriented approaches to mitigating risks. What are the strengths and weaknesses of both techniques? With which do you most resonate? How might you contribute to the development of more effective techniques at your institution?
- In the context of the ICU environment—high acuity patients; busy; noisy; multiple teams; and shared decision making—what steps can you take to minimise error or mistakes in your work?

Aftercare

Staff [aftercare] is almost non-existent when it comes to medical. I think the aftercare of patients is usually fine—I think that's fine. I mean they're still here if they survive. They're still here, so we are still looking after them medically, and bio-socially and so forth, if you like… Aftercare of families…so we do open disclose. Which I think is important… In terms of staff aftercare… Certainly for medical, that's close to non-existent.

- Although best practice in self-care would advocate the taking of some time to process traumatic events such as the death of a patient, the ICU is a busy place where healthcare providers are often required to move quickly from one acute case to the next, without immediate reflection. Is this something that you anticipated?
- The quote above suggests that aftercare programs are 'non-existent'. Do you perceive this as true also, or do you believe that this may simply be due to lack of awareness or a mix of both?
- Given that the nature of the environment may not afford you the time to process an event in the moment, what plans can you put in place to ensure you take time and space to do this as soon as you can?
- Is there a quiet go-to place within your institution?
- Do you know the processes and resources available to you within your institution to access confidential informal and formal support if it was needed for yourself or someone you know?
- In addition, consider resources that may be available outside your institution. What options might exist?
- An important consideration is the impact that self-care processes can have on family and friends. In your experience so far, have family and friends been able to effectively serve as sounding boards for self-care? Do you think this process can remain effective over the long term? Why or why not?
- Consider now the staff with which you work. What do you think their aftercare needs might be? What programs might be put in place—for example, post-event debriefing or pastoral care—to assist in team aftercare? How might you become involved with such programs?

Conclusion

As the above quotes illustrate, the ICU environment contains a diverse array of stressors. From the high-stakes decisions required to help each patient heal through the social difficulties created by the presence of multiple consulting services, intensivists often need to be all things to all people but have little time to consider the effects of this on their own resilience and emotional health. In situations such as this, opportunities to mentally rehearse potential responses and approaches can often make the difference between effective and ineffective management. Additionally, by considering potential positive coping mechanisms well ahead of time, intensivists can strengthen the resolve needed to engage these mechanisms during difficulty. The 'sea' of an intensivists career will be filled with moments of violent storms alongside blissful periods with tranquil waters. There will be shark attacks one moment and schools of playful dolphins the next. It is my hope that the thought exercises outlined above can provide a rubric for those wishing to engage in this process and can assist intensivists in training as they attempt to gain the skills needed to maintain a long, healthy and fruitful career.

Chapter 9
Nearly Drowning, Diagnosing Bias: Contemplating Societal Biases

Laura Hawryluck (iD)

> *You don't drown by falling in the water; you drown by staying there.*
>
> —Edwin Louis Cole

There are many things you don't get taught in medical school or in the long years of residency or fellowships. Some of the most challenging issues to deal with, no matter your stage of career, are those of societal biases, discrimination on any basis and flat-out racism. We have used the allegory of 'nearly drowning' for this chapter because, in the professional context, these societal biases may be expressed towards ICU physicians at a time when they are doing their utmost to stabilize a life-threatening illness, when they have succeeded in saving a patient's life or when they must explain that medical science is unable to prevent a patient from dying. In the ICU, sometimes such comments are made more 'innocently', almost inadvertently, as an expression of surprise or without thought, awareness and/or recognition. Sometimes such comments are expressed deliberately, a reflection of long-held hateful or racist beliefs and values, with a request to have a physician or a member of the healthcare team removed from providing much needed care. Sometimes they are also made quite deliberately and used to discredit or even belittle the physician whose role is to convey bad news or to engage in very difficult discussions about someone's condition. Sometimes the ICU physician may witness such comments being made about one of their inter-professional team members, their colleagues or, even in more relaxed social contexts. Such comments both wound and haunt. They threaten to drown therapeutic relationships between patients, families, physicians and team members at a time when this relationship is most needed. They make ICU physicians (and any others on the receiving end of such comments) feel misunderstood, isolated and alone in both their professional and personal lives. Yet rarely do

L. Hawryluck (✉)
Inter Divisional Department of Intensive Care, Toronto Western Hospital,
Toronto, ON, Canada
e-mail: Laura.Hawryluck@uhn.ca

we teach or mentor our trainees and colleagues on how to address or stand up for each other when witnessing such comments. This chapter offers an allegorical lifebuoy.

A fundamental tenet of medicine is that those in need of help are to be treated equally, with equity when needed, and physicians ought to meet and accept people as they are, without passing judgement and without making them feel less valued or deserving of empathy and care. But what happens when you witness a professional colleague, a friend even, make a derogatory comment about or, even to a patient or their family? What happens when you say something biased, discriminatory or even racist? Often this gets ascribed to being 'burnt out', 'letting off stress' or struggling with professional and/or personal obligations. Healthcare workers are people too. They are products of their upbringings and society. Are they truly immune to societal biases? Can they truly isolate their personal beliefs from their professional obligations every single time they need to? What does it mean or say about you, your colleague or friend if they express such biases when someone is in need and vulnerable? How do you address such comments and behaviours? The following quotations and questions will promote both self-reflection and discussion of some of the most challenging moments in an ICU physician's personal and professional life.

Perception of Judgement Towards Healthcare Workers from People Outside of Medicine

I think one of the hardest things is how you interact with the mother who says, "Oh, what you do for a living"? And if you… I frequently hedge and tell them that I am a pediatrician who works in the hospital. Or I just tell them I work at the children's hospital. Because that, I think… It makes people very aghast that you would choose to do this work. And I think that's one of the hardest things. Like, "How can you…" "I couldn't do that…" "That would break my heart, how can you work in that kind of environment?' Almost like, 'How can you be a person that does that"? "Don't you have feelings"? The most frequent thing that people say is "I could never do that, because I love children too much".

- Society has historically held doctors in high regard though this is changing to some extent. Do you believe there are differences in how ICU doctors are perceived compared with others? Are they positive or negative? Do they change based on world or local news events? What influences these changes in perceptions in your experiences and/or reflections?
- Do you hesitate to describe what you do? If yes, what drives this reluctance?
- How do you usually describe what you do? Do you ever feel you need to prevaricate and/or defend being an ICU physician, and if so, why?
- Do you feel that people make assumptions that you are not a physician (based on characteristics you can't change) but that you must instead be a member of the inter-professional ICU team? If yes, how do you handle such assumptions?

- What do you think your response might be if someone was to judge you negatively or, perceive you as only having an increased capacity to inflict pain or suffering on your patients in the ICU or as only prolonging their life on machines?
- How do you respond to comments such as 'Oh…. I wouldn't want to live *that* way'?
- What are the emotional and psychological impacts you experience when people make negative comments on what you do? Do they have the power to wound you? Do you feel you have acquired skills in working with people that help you cope?
- The COVID-19 pandemic shone a light on the intensive care environment, but past the ventilators and the acuity, do you think that people really understand what it is that you and your team do?
  What can you do in your everyday work to generate understanding, acceptance and appreciation of your ICU facility, its staff and the work it undertakes among the people in your life and in your wider community?

Perception of Discrimination Towards Healthcare Workers from Other Teams Based Upon Gender—Mutual Respect

I think a lot of it comes down to dealing with interactions with other treating teams – particularly some other treating teams that have a heavier male-bias to them – are or can be dismissive and not take the female intensivist with the same gravitas as they would … an older grey-haired male intensivist. I think that's a major challenge… It's very interesting and a lot of that subconscious bias that occurs in potential distribution of workloads and responsibilities, and the potential impact of (having) children on career progression are significant.

One of the most stressful things (as a female) is just the fight to be taken seriously by older male colleagues. You know, not just necessarily in intensive care, but across the board. …You know a lot of people have actually no insight or respect for your expertise… and you do get a bit of that from the male junior doctors as well.

- Medicine as a reflection of society has traditionally been male dominated, and though this is changing, it still holds true in many fields especially in ones to which more power is ascribed. Moreover, it is not only gender identification/expression and sexual orientation that may influence how seriously you are perceived or how seriously you are taken by other colleagues and/or team members, whether they are on your ICU team or another healthcare team. How do you think you might feel about not being taken seriously by a colleague—senior or not—based on *who* you are?
- If you felt someone was being disrespectful or dismissive of your opinion or perspective based on personal characteristics you can't change, would you address it in the moment or follow up with them later?

- Would your approach change if such discrimination events were perpetuated by a more senior colleague, one in a position of power, one otherwise highly respected as compared with a junior colleague or a trainee? If yes how?
- How would you communicate your concerns? What do you think would be effective? What would you do if it didn't work?
- Sometimes our past experiences, whether professional or personal, impact the lens through which current or future experiences are interpreted. Do you think this has ever happened to you?
- If your perception of discrimination within the relationship continued, was spread to others and/or escalated, how would you manage it? What do you think would be effective? What would you do if it didn't work?
- What if you were a bystander to this behaviour, whereby a colleague of yours was being disrespected? How would you act/react?
- Who have you turned to, and/or who would you turn to for help in processing the emotional and psychological impact of such events? What would be most helpful to you in coping with such situations?
- If you witnessed such events, how would they change how you interacted with the perpetrator of the discrimination in the future?
- What does allyship or advocacy mean in such contexts?
- How can you promote a healthy, respectful work environment?
- Are you aware of how you would lodge a complaint with your institution related to this sort of behaviour?
- Have you ever left a hospital because this was happening? Have you or do you know of anyone who has sought legal advice because of such events?

Perception of Discrimination Towards Healthcare Workers from Patients and their Families Based Upon Gender— Women Presumed to Be Nurses

I've had a family member… She liked me; she gave me a card; I think I still have it; she gave me a card that said, "Thank you for being such a great head nurse". I took care of her kid for like, two weeks [as an intensivist].

I've had ones where we walk in the room and there is an assumption that's been made about me already – that I'm the nurse who is following the doctor. So, you kind of just have to say, it's pleasantly surprising if it doesn't happen….

- Have you ever been mistaken for one over the other, or have you witnessed a colleague being misidentified?
- What sort of feelings have/would go through your head if you realised that for some time a patient or their family have had this role confusion?
- Are there patient/family factors that would make you more of less upset regarding such role confusion, for example, age, gender, ethnicity, time spent with them, or scope/intensity of interactions?

- Do you feel it is important to correct the mistake, and if so, why?
- How do/did you address the incorrect presumption?
- How do such events affect the therapeutic relationship?
- How would you discuss such an event with a student/trainee or colleague that witnessed it? How would you prepare them for and mentor them through a similar event happening to them?
- What do you think could help prevent such role confusion and/or biases?

Perception of Discrimination Towards Healthcare Workers from Patients and Their Families Based Upon Gender—Men Presumed to Be Directing Care

She was like my hero… my absolute hero…. because she was incredible, and I was like "I want to be 1/10 of what you are…" And when I would be at a bedside, and she would be telling the family like "what was up", and they'd be looking at me and like (asking), "so do you agree with that"? She would throw it all in… "Why don't you tell them what you think, sport?" and it just became a problem for me. I mean she knew enough… Her emotional intelligence was high enough to know, you know… "I'm not gonna pick a fight with (this) family… Like, no one is at fault here, this is just a broken part of society… This person wasn't being malicious…".

- The assignment of incorrect role identity to healthcare workers by stakeholders is common. Role assumptions can be grounded in several factors: age, appearance, clothing, gender/ gender expression, ethnicity and medical fields, to name but a few. How such events handled by those involved may affect how they are perceived more broadly, the quality and nature of their professional, mentoring and educational relationships moving forward. Have you ever witnessed or created an event such as the one described?
- Do you feel that you, as a staff intensivist, have ever displaced your emotional/ psychological reaction and frustrations to the innocent bystander colleague or trainee/student? Have you ever witnessed such a response?
- Imagine yourself to be the person presumed by the patient to be in charge. It's awkward. What would you do? What do you say, and to whom? And when do you do these things?
- Now imagine yourself to be the person presumed by the patient to be junior, when you are in fact directing care. It's awkward too. What would do you do? What do you say, and to whom? And when do you do these things?
- Many patients meet a lot of healthcare professionals during a hospital stay. Should there be a better approach to helping patients/families understand who is who? What would that look like?
- Are there other root causes of role and responsibility misidentification that you can think of?

Perception of Discrimination Towards Healthcare Workers from Patients and Their Families Based Upon Their Age or Level of Experience

Occasionally, a family will "fire" a care giver – usually a medical student, a new nurse or a young resident that they perceive is a "weak link" in their child's care. Families that struggle in academic environments will share that they "don't want people learning on their children" and/or "practicing on them". They want to be able to speak to the individual directing their child's care and struggle with the hierarchy that involves learners gathering the information and more senior providers synthesizing and integrating the story/data to develop a plan… They need to know that the youngest members of the team or the members of the team that appear to ask the most questions and have the fewest answers, often are the ones that are asking the questions that make us all think harder and in more detail about the patient at hand.

- As life-long learners, we are all novice learners of something. Have you ever experienced requests to not have students or trainees involved in care?
- What would be some ways to reassure our patients and their families that trainees or students will offer quality and appropriately supervised healthcare?
- Consider a patient who is refusing to be treated by a trainee. How would you explore their concerns, and how might you frame your response? Practice your conversation with them out aloud.
- How have/would you explain to the trainee that the patient or their family doesn't want them involved in their care? If the students/trainees were initially involved, how would you explain to a student/trainee that the patient or their family *no longer* wants them involved in their care?
- How would you support and mentor a student/trainee who has been told directly by a patient or their family that they do not want them participating in their care?
- If you were the supervising ICU physician in such a situation when an agreement was reached that they would participate in care, would you change how you provide care to such a patient or their family? How you supervise your team? If yes, how and why?
- If you were the student/trainee in such a situation when an agreement was reached that they would participate in care, would you change how you provide care to such a patient or their family? If yes, how and why?
- If you receive negative feedback about students and trainees in such situations, when an agreement was reached that they would participate in care, how do you assess if it is accurate and free of bias or prejudice?
- If you were the student/trainee in such a situation when an agreement was reached that they would participate in care, how do you respond to such feedback? Would you perceive any value in such feedback? Would it provide a learning opportunity?
- What about if you were that student/trainee, how might you respond in terms of how you would introduce yourself to the next patient you are asked to manage?

- What would happen if an error event had occurred after you reached an agreement that the student/trainee would participate in the patient's care after the initial request that they not do so? How you support and mentor the students/trainees through an error event in such situations?
- Do you feel that such requests add to any stress and anxiety you may feel as an ICU physician in a teaching role?

Perception of Bias Impacting Trajectory of the Patient Journey Based on Religious Beliefs

A 92-year-old Orthodox Jewish man with extensive bowel carcinoma was being managed in the intensive care after a laparotomy for bowel perforation with extensive faecal soiling of the peritoneal cavity, sepsis and multiple organ failure. After explaining the gravity of the situation and the slim chance of survival, the son said: "I hear and understand what you are saying, but we put our hope and trust in God. He decides who lives and dies, and not you. Even suffering has a value, as long as life is preserved. Continue full support".

- Sometimes a poor patient prognosis is clear, and equally clear is that there are no further treatments that will be able to change the outcome. Despite this, life support is continued—regardless of discussions that it will only prolong the patient's death and add to their suffering. In some instances, this continuation is due to personal or religious beliefs of the patient and/or their family and in others due to distrust or disbelief of the prognosis or distrust of/conflict with the healthcare system and/or the past or current healthcare teams. Sometimes it's the expressed hope for 'a miracle' that will happen if treatments are continued. Yet medical science was never intended to hurt more than it helps, nor was it intended to be a tool to only cause harm, create or add to suffering. When ICU care is continued when it can no longer help, ongoing discussions of treatment goals and limitations that should be placed on ongoing treatments are draining and distressing for all involved. When confronted by such decisions or insistence on continuing treatments that can no longer help, how do you react? Do you find it difficult to maintain a therapeutic relationship with patients and families in such circumstances?
- Do you revisit this discussion, and if so, how regularly? Are such repeated discussions helpful, or do they cause conflicts with people increasingly entrenched in their positions? What do you feel would help maintain communication and the therapeutic relationship?
- Have you ever refused to continue providing care to patients in such situations? Have you witnessed a colleague express such a refusal?
- Do you feel it is possible to limit care, for example, its escalation, without the family's consent and/or without their knowledge? What is the role of a physician's fiduciary duties in such circumstances?

- Have you or your team ever changed how you interact with the family in ways that ensure the family has a clearer 'understanding' of how much suffering the patient is experiencing?
- What do you do if you witness your team members ensuring the family 'understands' just what the patient is going through?
- Have you ever made negative, derogatory or disrespectful comments to your team members about the patient or their family's beliefs and their wish to continue treatment? What would be a better approach to help yourself and the team cope and navigate such situations?
- In your country and within your facility, is it possible to withdraw care without the family's consent? What, if any legal recourses, do you have to advocate for your patient and prevent causing more suffering? Have you ever engaged with the legal system in such situations? Why or why not?
- Do such requests to continue when ICU treatments can no longer help impact how you approach the next patient/family from same religious, belief system or cultural background?
- Do you feel such requests to continue negatively impact your team's approach to subsequent patients and families from same religious, belief system or cultural background? What steps could you take that would help you prevent or mitigate this impact?

Perception of Bias Impacting Patient Safety Based on Religious Beliefs

Women could only be examined with a male family member as a witness in the room. As such they would leave their abayas on and we would examine them under their clothes. One teenage girl had gone to get an ECG (Electrocardiogram): a process whereby small circular stickers with a clip in the centre are put on key areas of the chest, electrical leads are attached to them and the electrical impulse of the heart's conduction system is studied. After her ECG, she was asked to remove her stickers, and she did so. No one else took them off because we didn't want to expose her or feel for the stickers under her abaya. Later on in the day it was determined that she needed an MRI (Magnetic Resonance Imaging). Because the centre of the sticker is metal, it heats up in an MRI scanner and the magnet will pull the metal to it, pulling the skin with it. The young woman sustained a burn and a tissue tear when her ECG sticker was pulled off during the MRI. I remember the women on the team felt great shame that we had not examined her before going into the MRI scanner and that we had provided her with "less than" care because of modesty and we failed to provide her with the medicine she deserved.

- Reflecting on some of the situations that you may have encountered, how have you attempted to balance respect with your obligations to disclose information and maintain patient safety?

- How do you think you would respond to this scenario in terms of your conversation with the patient and her family after this event that would perhaps help improve the balance between respect and safety in future healthcare encounters?
- Have you ever felt frustrations or other negative reactions towards patients who 'let' religious/cultural/personal beliefs impact their interactions with physicians and healthcare teams? How has this impacted your therapeutic relationship?
- Have you ever witnessed a healthcare professional struggling with their own reaction to such situations? Do you feel their reaction impacted the care they provided to the patient? How would you handle this situation?
- Have you ever made negative, derogatory or disrespectful comments to your team members about the patient's or their family's beliefs/requests in such situations? What would be a better approach to help yourself and the team cope and navigate such situations?
- How would you respond if you witness a colleague making negative comments in such situations?
- What role do such patient care events and your responses to them play in the propagation of biases towards colleagues and team members who may be from the same faith or cultural background? In the creation of a safe and welcoming workspace, where diversity is welcome and celebrated?

Perception of Negative Discrimination Towards Patients and Their Families Based Upon Race or Socioeconomic Factors

Negative experiences are fuelled by parental distrust of the medical system in general. We had a patient who came in after a terrible car accident, who was clearly going to die. They had an arrest at the scene, but were resuscitated here, and were dying. And the family had such a deep distrust of the medical system. They thought that because they were poor and black, that they would not receive the same medical care as another family would. And so it took quite a long time to build enough trust to even get them to a point where they could understand that their child had died because of a severe brain injury. It was a tough situation.

The opposite of poverty isn't wealth; the opposite of poverty is justice. We practice in a system where poor people do not always get the same care as their wealthier counterparts.

- Socioeconomic status can be a barrier to the delivery of optimal healthcare in so many ways, and the past experiences people have will always influence their current perceptions. Most people might presume that the life of a doctor is one of relative privilege and that they came from a life of privilege. The issue for many healthcare providers is, on the one hand, that might be true and they may struggle to use their lived experiences as a basis upon which to build empathy. On the other hand, if they come from a more modest or poor socioeconomical background and can relate to financial struggles, their patients may not believe this to be true. In either case the delivery of optimal healthcare may be compromised. Moreover, many physicians have witnessed that sometimes there is a very real impact of socioeconomic status on patient care. Imagine you come from a family whose background is within a racial minority and that, in your past, you have experienced disrespectful behaviours from healthcare professionals that you perceive were racially discriminatory. What mindset do you bring to an emergent scenario where you are told the outcome for your family member looks grim?

- Have you ever been in a situation where the patient or family perceived you were biased? What happened? How did you deal with their reactions and feedback?
- Have you ever witnessed a colleague, student or trainee express a bias or discriminatory comments or behaviour? How have you handled such situations? What could you do differently in the future?
- What do you think might help you to believe that the situation being relayed to you is free from bias or discrimination?
- Are you aware of any liaison services within the healthcare system that may help build trust and foster communications? What obstacles if any exist in getting them engaged? What could help improve the help they provide?
- Trust is earned. As the team leader, how might you engender trust that best care is being administered and that opinions are independent of your background financial status or racial/ethnic/cultural, gender identity or expression?
- Do you believe and make efforts and take steps to ensure the healthcare you provide is equitable? What steps do you take to mentor and teach such an approach to healthcare?
- What steps can you take to ensure such biases are not propagated in healthcare? What steps do you feel the healthcare system can/should take as it strives to help address such issues?
- What can you do to build trust within the communities you serve?

Perception of Positive Discrimination Towards Patients and their Families Based Upon Socioeconomic Factors

The patients are labelled as VIP – "Very Important" – because of their family's wealth, prestige or role within the community. These are families we feel compelled to over communicate with. This often presents as a burden in that multiple detailed conversations need to be sure that the VIP family understands the treatment plan being outlined and why certain labs, painful procedures, interventions need to be done… there are (also) times when care teams resent the VIP patients: they are perceived to "leapfrog" over others for appointments and specialist attention.

- There is an overarching theme here as to whether 'very important' people (VIP) should be given any concessions in the delivery of healthcare, and there may be arguments for and against. VIPs may also include other healthcare professionals (or members of their families) who may or may not work within your own hospital. The provision of care to VIPs may be clouded by a perceived or real sense of entitlement, pressures for senior colleagues or hospital administrators to ensure the care and support to the patient and family are particularly diligent or even above and beyond what is required. There may also be pressure by senior colleagues or hospital administrators to provide them with updated, detailed information on the patient's progress. Such pressures and tensions may create unnecessary additional stress and anxiety, and the added attention may actually detract from the quality and effectiveness of the care itself. Furthermore, resentment and frustrations may arise when the attention that is being demanded, whether by the patient, family, or hospital, detracts from the very real need to care for others, many of whom may be sicker and need more time and focus than the VIP.
- Have you ever cared for a VIP patient? Did you experience some of the negative aspects as described in this quote? How did you handle this situation?
- Knowing that these features are usually recurrent in the care of such patients, what are the things you might put in place to optimise both communication and care?
- How would/have you set boundaries to maintain the VIP patient's right to privacy and confidentiality? What happens when you are confronting breaches in such care principles from people with power over you and/or from people who ought to know better?
- How do you handle VIPs who may be biased against the ICU care delivery (e.g., the inclusion of students, trainees and inter-professional team members in rounds and in communications)?
- How do you cope with VIPs when they disagree with treatments not being offered or with limitations placed on treatment escalation? Is your approach different when compared with other patients? What would help improve such discussions?
- Have you ever experienced a highly ranked hospital administrator or senior colleague pulling you aside to express that the care you provide could have a positive impact on the hospital—either on a reputational basis or through future donations/funding—if all goes well. How would you respond to such a statement? Would this be a source of stress and how would you manage this?
- Have you ever consulted with another colleague on how to cope with a VIP or been asked for advice? What do you feel would be helpful to know?
- Do you ever feel frustrated and challenged when treating another physician who does literature searches on their diagnosis and potential treatment options? Why do you think they do such searches? Have you as a physician or healthcare worker ever been a patient? How did you cope/react to being on the other side of the bed?

- How do you respond to VIP people (with medical training or without) who bring medical literature or Google searches to your attention and want to engage in a detailed debate? What could you do that would help improve such interactions?
- When VIP people offer to harness or obtain scarcer resources by 'making phone calls' to either speed the availability of needed imaging, how do you react? Do such offers give rise to any negative feelings towards the VIP patient or family?

Bias Towards Patient and Their Family from the Healthcare Team Based on Their Frequency of Readmission

The reality of being an intensivist is that as medicine improves our ability to sustain life, it also sometimes creates a population of extremely fragile and often technology-dependent patients that can have a "revolving door" of ICU needs. These patients and their accompanying families come tethered to their past hospitalizations, for better or worse. Doctors can remember past arguments, demands, or social dysfunctions. In the pediatric ICU, for example, families of chronically ill children are asked to become providers of 24/7 nursing care when they bring their child home, but the chronic physical and emotional strain of this reality is something that the ICU doctor is insulated from…until readmission(s), when a medically fragile patient living in poverty needs ICU-level care repeatedly after contracting bacterial or viral infections. These patients embody the frustrating reality that areas of a doctor's concern and areas that they can impact are not the same.

I mean, this patient has literally come in every several months since being born. He has a tracheostomy, is on a ventilator at home, and ongoing severe seizures, so we kind of expect him to need care on a pretty frequent basis, especially during respiratory season, but each time he comes in he looks a little worse, a little more cachectic. I know it must be hard to care for him at home, but it's hard not to form negative opinions about the family, especially given how defensive confrontational they are about his home care. It makes us want to avoid talking to them when he is admitted, but that is just not good for care. It's a struggle.

- Many families of chronically critically ill patients want to continue caring for them at home, despite the physicians' and healthcare teams very open and transparent discussion of what the patient's life would look like, the risks and complications, the challenges—if not impossibility of being a caregiver 24/7—and the reality of insufficient community resources being available to support them in such a role. Sometimes when families experience the realities of the demands of such care, it is clear they can't cope despite their best intentions and the patient gets re-admitted in an increasingly deteriorating state. Such deteriorations are understandable yet can be frustrating to cope with when the family is hypervigilant in hospital, demanding that everything be fixed (even when it can't) and insists on once again returning home against medical advice. It can also be frustrating when families insist on continuing even though the patient's quality of life is clearly worsening and their end of life is is nearing . Such family insistence on continuing life-saving care may be grounded in the perception that the patient enjoys interactions with their loved ones and yet, when in hospital, the family 'disappears' and is never present. In other situations, the family may succeed in providing exemplary care at home, better than can be achieved in hospital, yet it is clear to the physician and healthcare team that the family is exhausted and the patient is nevertheless continuing to deteriorate. Have you ever considered that physicians or members of the ICU team may have conscious and subconscious biases towards the chronically critically ill patients and their quality of life, the resources required to care for them, the values/beliefs and judgment of their families?

- Have you ever had a negative reaction to hearing that a chronically critically ill patient has been brought to the ED and will likely require ICU admission?
- What do you feel drives the negative reactions or biases that ICU physicians and teams may feel towards these patients and their families? Are such reactions driven by considerations of perceived quality of life? By past conflicts while in the acute stages of critical illness? Are chronically critically ill patients perceived as a failure of acute ICU care?
- Have you ever felt that the quality of care you have provided to such patients was not up to your usual standards? What do you feel impacted the care you provided?
- How have you responded to witnessing negative comments or biased comments from your colleagues or team members and their impact on the care of chronically critically ill patients?
- Have you witnessed ICU team members refuse to provide care to such patients? Have you experienced them making comments that suggest they feel such patients are not 'real ICU patients' or in some way not deserving of ICU care?
- Is an ICU ever a destination for 'respite' care for a family who desperately needs a relief from caring for a loved one on a home ventilator? Should/could there be a way for some ICUs to provide respite care? What would that look like?

Biases Towards Those Struggling with Mental Health Problems, Addictions, Self-Harming

The call usually comes in from the Emergency Department. 'We are calling about a "frequent flyer"…. They are an indigenous patient who presents every few weeks intoxicated. They are a known cocaine and fentanyl user…. Often, they come to the ED and we let them sleep it off and they leave AMA (against medical advice) to the shelter to use some more. This time they presented so obtunded we had to intubate…. Oh, and it's not clear if they got into a fight with one of their "friends", they have a black eye and some bruises. I don't think they are seriously hurt though'. I just feel this is SO wrong – the language and description sets up anchoring biases about what has actually happened to this patient…. On more than one occasion, it caused a delay in diagnosing a life-threatening problem… an intracranial bleed… or other injuries that needed urgent treatment.

Sometimes I feel physicians and healthcare teams give up on patients before they even start trying to help them. I often get told why are you even bothering trying to get Addiction Services involved …why ask social work to explore community supports and housing. They are just going to use again. It's a waste of time. I often get told similar things when treating patients with difficult to control mental health illnesses who repeatedly attempt to self-harm…. Its only going to keep happening. Why are you wasting your time? But…. What kind of doctor, what kind of person, would I be if I didn't try to help?

- Caring for those who are struggling with chronic mental health illnesses including addiction can be very challenging as they often require repeated admissions, often self-treat with polysubstance use and often engage in self-harm. They are commonly marginally housed, struggle with poor hygiene and general health and struggle from a socioeconomic perspective. They are vulnerable to inter-personal violence and abuse be it emotional, psychological, physical and sexual in nature. Sometimes the elderly in society, those living in long-term care facilities, are also seen through a similar lens—they are 'old', 'what do you expect?, they are only going to get re-admitted, they are only going to die', 'they have advanced dementia, they have no quality of life' or other comments such as 'Don't go out of your way, this is all that can be expected from long term care homes… it's up to the family to complain'. Have you ever stopped to think of the contrast between the care provided to those with mental illness, polysubstance use, self-harming behaviours and VIP people?
- What about when you are asked to care for the elderly needing recurrent admissions. What differences in care do they experience? How may their past healthcare experiences impact their therapeutic relationship with you as a physician? Their family's initial reaction to you and their relationship with you as a physician?
- Have you ever been told that you are wasting your time trying to help, advocate and achieve some change in level of community supports for such patients? Do you feel this is an expression of bias? How have you felt/responded?
- Have you ever witnessed expressions of covert or overt bias and discrimination towards such patients? Who, in your experiences, have you heard such comments from? Have such comments changed your perception of that physician/ healthcare team member as a professional and/or as a person?
- How would you respond to people who express such biases? Would you do so privately or publicly, and what would determine the timing of your response?
- Would your response to such biases and or discriminatory behaviours change if you witnessed it being done by a colleague within the ICU as compared to one working in another department or hospital ward?

- Have you experienced or could you imagine missed diagnosis events that you attribute to assumptions made based on the patient's chronic health problems? What happened? How might this have been prevented?
- If you have tried to provide care and gone above and beyond in advocating for the patient in an attempt to provide them with some stability and opportunities to improve their health, were these successful? Would you try to help in this way again- why or why not? What did you learn?

Criminal Perpetrators—Adults and Children

We had a particularly brutal murder complicated by self-inflicted injuries (by the accused) to try and deflect the blame, and both patients were being treated in the resus area together … the perpetrator survived, and the victim didn't. There was a lot of talk around why we were spending so much time on the perpetrator and not leaving him alone while we dealt with the victim….

The ones [child abuse cases] that need intensive care – they are abusive head injuries that occur in infancy. And I have two responses. One is the sadness of "How you could do this to a kid"? The other is anger. Just being angry at the perpetrator, whoever that may be. In fact, my response is, when I hear that visitor restrictions preclude anybody from being at the child's bedside for the first couple of days - I go, "Thank God I don't have to actually look at somebody in the eye and comfort them about their child when I think there's a good chance that they were the ones that inflicted the injuries". At the same time, it's not my job to figure out who did it, my job is to just identify it and pass it on to the police and let them do their investigation. And so, there's a part of me that tries not to be judgemental, but it's also hard not to be.

- In healthcare, we are often faced with the sequelae of violence and trauma secondary to criminal behaviour of one kind or another. Such events include those of intimate partner violence, elder and child abuse. In the ICU, it is the victims that are most often in need of care. Their injuries can be horrific, difficult to understand with respect to how they could be inflicted on another human being and, once seen, unable to be unseen. They can destroy our belief in humanity. Sometimes they result in significant long-term morbidities, and sometimes they are lethal. Sometimes the patient has injuries that the physician feels are a result of assault and interpersonal violence, yet the justice system is unaware and uninvolved of the situation. Sometimes the suspicion is that the perpetrator may be the person who would normally be in the surrogate decision-maker role or someone who was in a caregiver role. Have you ever had to provide care for a patient whose injuries are the result of interpersonal violence? How has this affected the care you provide? Does it change the way you communicate with them and/or their families?

- Have you ever felt more concerned about the pain and suffering that the care you provide in the ICU may cause such patients who have already been hurt by someone?
- Do you feel/can you imagine feeling that you have to provide more care, go beyond any limits you would normally place on treatment escalation as a way of 'righting the wrong'?
- Have you ever felt it hard to control how you feel towards the perpetrator? Towards anyone else in the patient's life that you feel could have prevented these events? How have you managed/coped with such feelings? What was helpful?
- If you have a colleague, team member, student or trainee struggling with how they feel, what guidance would you provide to help them navigate this situation?
- Have you ever cared for a patient injured by an intimate partner, and had that patient recover only to refuse to press charges? How did you manage this situation?
- Have you ever felt or witnessed someone expressing that a patient injured by an intimate partner 'should just leave' and because they should have known this would happen? How have you reflected on such feelings and/or responded if you have witnessed such comments?
- Have you ever had to provide care for a patient whose injuries you suspect are the result of interpersonal violence, yet the police are not involved?
- Do you think you would react/feel differently if the patient was an adult as compared to a child?
- If the patient was a child and the suspected or confirmed abuser a parent or someone who had access to the child through a parent, would that change how you would interact with them (i.e. the one who did not directly inflict the abuse)?
- Have you thought about how you are going to feel providing care to a family member who you understand to be the main suspect in a criminal event that has resulted in your patient's admission? Would it change how you provide care or how you communicate?
- How do you imagine your team will respond to providing care to a suspected perpetrator? Do you think any members would take umbrage with a perpetrator receiving more attention/care that the person they harmed if such care was warranted?
- What behaviours will you encourage your team to display towards a suspected perpetrator?
- There may also be legal proceedings in which you are required to participate. Can you imagine how your feelings may affect how you would document in the chart and how you would subsequently provide your medical evidence in court if required? Would it change how openly you would communicate with the police?

Conclusion

We all view the world, its events and its people, through our own lens. This lens has been shaped by how we were nurtured (or not), our upbringing (including but not limited to our home environments, our families, our teachers), what we have experienced, what we have witnessed, what we have read, the people in our lives, our reactions and those of others to life events and the lessons learned. Equally important, yet perhaps somewhat overlooked in the shaping of our lens, is our state of health, the illnesses we have experienced or witnessed and the caring (or not) that was received. Seeing the world through different lenses, in other words having inherent biases, is not a negative—in fact the diversity that different views, cultures, beliefs and perceptions bring can be enriching and can result in new ideas, innovations and better ways to live. Yet when these biases create negative perceptions, discriminate, or develop notions that people have less worth than others, that they are less worthy of healthcare when in need or that its acceptable that they have less access to care readily available to others, it's not okay. Being more aware of one's own lens can help mitigate its real or potential negative impact on the lives of others, in particular for some of the most vulnerable of all: those with a life-threatening illness. It is my hope the scenarios discussed here, which represent only some of the moments in which caution is required, will help broaden that lens and will promote clarity when close focus is so needed. For isn't the most important question of all: what does it mean to you to share a common humanity?

Chapter 10
Swimming in New Waters: Contemplating the ICU Environment after a Pandemic

Kenneth Remy and Qalab Abbas

> *What world lies beyond that stormy sea I do not know, but every ocean has a distant shore, and I shall reach it.*
>
> —Cesare Pavese

The early months of 2020 marked the onset of a global crisis that reshaped our society and tested the very limits of human resilience. The COVID-19 pandemic was a defining chapter in the lives and careers of intensive care doctors all over the world. It tested their limits as physicians, scientists, and human beings. It reinforced the importance of compassion, resilience, and adaptability in the face of unprecedented challenges. It also highlighted the power of communication—and miscommunication.

Although this time was immensely uncertain and stressful, it provided us with the opportunity to adapt to a new normal and brought many silver linings into our personal and professional lives. We believe that this pandemic tested us and made us more adaptable, resilient, and empathetic. We are grateful to our hospitals, universities, mentors, patients, and our families for embarking on and surviving this journey with us.

In the end, the pandemic was not just about a virus. It was about people—the patients who fought valiantly, the families who grieved, and the healthcare workers who gave everything they had. It was about humanity at its most vulnerable and its most courageous. And it was about the enduring hope that even in the darkest times, we can find a way forward together.

K. Remy (✉)
University Hospitals of Cleveland/Case Western Reserve University Departments of Internal Medicine and Pediatric, Divisions of Pulmonary Critical Care and Pediatric Critical Care. The Blood, Heart, Lung, and Immunology Research Center of CWRU-UH,
Cleveland, OH, USA
e-mail: kenneth.remy@uhhospitals.org

Q. Abbas
Department of Pediatric and Child Health, Aga Khan University, Karachi, Pakistan
e-mail: qalab.abbas@aku.edu

© The Author(s), under exclusive license to Springer Nature Switzerland AG 2025
D. Dennis et al. (eds.), *Contemplating the Role of an Intensive Care Doctor*,
https://doi.org/10.1007/978-3-031-92766-9_10

In the chapter that follows, we describe our respective journey through the harrowing days of the pandemic, as two doctors, a world apart: one working in the United States (US) and one in Pakistan. As we move forward, the lessons of the pandemic must not be forgotten. From the need for robust public health infrastructure to the importance of global solidarity, COVID-19 revealed both our vulnerabilities and our strengths. For intensivists, it was a journey of profound loss and incredible resilience, one that will shape our approaches to medicine and life for years to come.

Through the Lens of a US-Based Physician-Scientist— Kenneth Remy

For me, an adult and pediatric ICU physician, it became a period defined by unrelenting challenges, heartbreaking losses, and profound lessons. Finding ways to "flatten the curve" when I was working for months without a day off, taking four showers a day, having many patients die daily, and then have individuals deny that COVID-19 was real or that wearing a mask could help were incredibly disheartening. The COVID-19 pandemic brought devastation to families and healthcare systems alike. It also thrust me into a dual role as both a clinician and a voice for public health. My experiences on the frontlines and the human stories that came with them continue to haunt and inspire me.

The Early Days: A Deluge of Uncertainty

As the first wave of COVID-19 reached the United States, the sheer magnitude of the crisis became evident almost overnight. In the ICUs where I worked, beds filled faster than we could discharge patients. What began as isolated cases rapidly escalated into an unrelenting torrent of critically ill individuals, each fighting a novel virus that was as unpredictable as it was deadly. We faced immense uncertainty about the virus itself. How did it spread so efficiently? Why did some patients deteriorate so rapidly while others remained asymptomatic? There was no playbook for what was to come, and the pressure to innovate, adapt, and provide answers weighed heavily on me and my colleagues.

The First Wave: A Relentless Battle

The first wave of the pandemic was defined by grueling work hours and an unrelenting sense of urgency. For 73 consecutive days, I worked in the ICU, where patient conditions often deteriorated despite our best efforts. Each shift brought new challenges—from severe equipment shortages to constantly evolving treatment protocols. But the most profound challenge was not medical—it was human. The ICU became a place of profound isolation, where visitors were prohibited to prevent the virus's spread. Patients fought their battles alone, unable to hold the hands of their loved ones in their final moments. In their absence, I became their surrogate family member, whispering reassurances, holding their hands as they took their last breaths, and bearing the unimaginable burden of calling families to deliver the devastating news. No amount of medical training could have prepared me for the emotional weight of those moments.

One case that remains etched in my memory is that of a father and son who were admitted to the ICU within days of each other. Both were critically ill, and despite our exhaustive efforts, neither survived. I still remember the anguish in their family's voices during those heart-wrenching phone calls—and the silence that followed their passing. These moments laid bare the virus's indiscriminate cruelty, leaving scars that no amount of time will erase.

Fear, Defiance, and the Clash of Public Perception

The pandemic exposed deep fractures in societal attitudes toward public health. Unlike countries where strict governmental mandates were swiftly enforced, the United States faced a unique duality: a population paralyzed by fear on one hand and emboldened by fierce independence and institutional distrust on the other. This defiance—expressed through mask resistance, vaccine scepticism, and outright denial of the virus's severity—contributed to surge volumes and preventable deaths. It was devastating to watch patients suffer from a disease they had refused to acknowledge just days before, their final words often filled with regret.

This clash between public perception and medical reality took a profound toll on MICU physicians. Each day, we walked into a warzone where science was questioned, even as we exhausted every option to save lives. The unknowns of the virus were daunting enough, but the weight of public doubt and misinformation compounded the emotional and professional toll. We battled not only a novel pathogen but also the exhaustion of constantly justifying our work—of pleading for preventive measures, only to be met with resistance.

The Unseen Cost: Physician Burnout and Career Dissatisfaction

The relentless waves of critically ill patients, the moral distress of witnessing preventable deaths, and the psychological toll of isolation led to an unprecedented level of burnout among MICU physicians. While some found renewed purpose in their work, many reconsidered their career paths entirely. The emotional strain of witnessing death after death, combined with the frustration of public noncompliance, eroded career satisfaction for countless intensivists. Some left critical care altogether. Others stayed, but not without deep scars—both personal and professional.

Despite the devastation, there were moments of resilience. Every patient who survived and reunited with their family reminded us why we continued fighting. But as we move forward, we must recognize that the pandemic fundamentally reshaped the MICU landscape, forcing us to reevaluate not only how we respond to crises but also how we support those who bear the brunt of these battles. The scars of this pandemic remain, and for many intensivists, the journey toward healing is far from over.

The Second Wave: A New Level of Exhaustion

As the second wave of COVID-19 surged, I once again found myself working over 2 consecutive months without a break. By then, we knew more about the virus—how it spread, how it ravaged the body, and how to keep our patients alive for just a little longer. But that knowledge did not lessen the burden. The emotional and physical toll of sustained crisis management was undeniable. Intubating over 300 patients was no longer just a clinical procedure; it was an intimate act of desperation—a race against time to save lives, knowing full well that for many, it would be in vain.

Some patients survived and went home to their families, a testament to the advancements we had made in care and sheer perseverance. Others did not. Each death felt like a personal failure, even when I knew we had done everything possible. The ICU had become a relentless theatre of life and death, where the stakes were always final. Husbands and wives died within hours of each other, leaving orphaned children behind. Young, seemingly healthy individuals succumbed to the virus, defying our understanding of risk factors. There was no justice, no predictability, only devastation.

A Crossroads for MICU Physicians: Fight or Flight

The unrelenting pressure shattered many of us. Some MICU physicians, drained beyond measure, walked away from the field entirely. The cost was too high—the sleepless nights, the crushing weight of loss, the futility of begging the public to take the virus seriously, only to see preventable deaths pile up. They left for less emotionally gruelling specialties or exited medicine altogether, unwilling to continue sacrificing their well-being in a system that often felt indifferent to their suffering.

Yet others, including myself, found their purpose strengthened. The burden of loss carved something deeper inside us—an unwavering resolve to stand in the gap for the dying, to fight harder, to heal not just bodies but the broken trust between medicine and society. We had looked into the abyss and did not turn away. We chose to stay.

For young doctors, the question is inevitable: What would you have done? If placed in the middle of an outbreak—whether Ebola, COVID-19, or the next pandemic—would you run toward it or away? Would you answer the call, knowing the personal cost? Medicine is not just a profession; it is a covenant with humanity. To be an ICU doctor is to accept that, at some point, you may be asked to risk your own life for another. That is the reality we faced. That is the reality you must be willing to face.

The Pandemic's Impact on My Life and Career

The pandemic changed me in ways I am still uncovering. It forced me to confront my own mortality, to find meaning in suffering, to navigate a world where science and misinformation waged war in the very spaces I was trying to save lives. It reinforced that the choice to stay in medicine—particularly in critical care—is not one of convenience. It is a calling. And it is not for everyone.

But for those who choose to stay, the rewards—while often overshadowed by the losses—are profound. To fight for the dying, to bear witness to both tragedy and survival, to stand in the chaos and still find purpose—this is what it means to be a MICU doctor. And despite everything, I would choose it all over again.

The Video That Spoke to the World

One moment that would forever shape my pandemic journey came during the second wave when I decided to create a public health video. The goal was simple: convey the seriousness of COVID-19 in a way that would resonate with the public. I recorded myself performing an intubation simulation, emphasizing the reality that many patients would face if they contracted the virus. The video, intended as a heartfelt plea for prevention, unexpectedly went viral, reaching over 200 million people worldwide. Media outlets from CNN to the BBC shared the footage, and suddenly, I found myself on a global stage.

Over the next few months, I gave more than 200 interviews to news outlets, discussing the importance of masks, social distancing, and vaccination. Public health experts, including Dr. Michael Osterholm, credited the video with contributing to what became known as "the Remy Effect"—a pivotal moment in "flattening the curve" by galvanizing public awareness and action. It was incredible to me how a simple video could inspire millions to act and save lives and how global outreach could touch those near and far.

Training for the Unknown

While I was in the spotlight, my primary focus remained on the ICU. As hospitals became overwhelmed, the demand for critical care expertise outpaced supply. During the first wave, I spearheaded efforts to train pediatric ICU doctors to care for adult patients, a task that required rapid upskill in ventilator management, sedation protocols, and end-of-life care for adults. This work extended far beyond my institution. Through virtual training sessions, I collaborated with healthcare professionals in resource-limited settings worldwide, sharing knowledge and strategies to combat the virus.

Science in the Time of Crisis

Even as I worked in the ICU, my laboratory pursued critical research. We were among the first to identify immune exhaustion as a key factor contributing to severe COVID-19 outcomes. Using patient samples collected during marathon shifts, we discovered how the virus hijacked the immune system, leaving patients vulnerable to secondary infections and organ failure. These findings, published in leading journals, informed clinical trials and therapeutic interventions, offered a glimmer of hope amidst the chaos.

Managing My Own Fears

The fear of contracting the virus lingered constantly in the back of my mind. Every intubation was performed with the knowledge that one wrong move could expose me or my loved ones to the disease. I feared bringing the virus home, infecting my family, and becoming another statistic. To mitigate the risk, I developed a meticulous routine: showering three to four times a day, disinfecting every item I carried, and driving through eerily empty streets on my way to work. The emptiness of the roads was haunting, a stark contrast to the chaos within the ICU.

Global Outreach and Resource-Limited Settings

While the pandemic overwhelmed well-resourced hospitals, its impact on resource-limited settings was catastrophic. Through virtual platforms, I provided consultation and education to healthcare providers in countries with limited access to ventilators, medications, and personal protective equipment. These sessions underscored the stark disparities in global healthcare systems and reinforced the need for international collaboration.

The Personal Cost

Beyond the professional demands, the pandemic exacted a personal toll. I missed countless family moments and carried the weight of my patients' stories home with me each night. The emotional scars of witnessing so much suffering and loss lingered long after my shifts ended. Yet, amidst the darkness, there were moments of hope. Seeing a patient recover and reunite with their family was a reminder of why we do what we do.

There were also times when my fears overwhelmed me. I lay awake at night, replaying the day's events and questioning whether I had done enough. The haunting images of patients struggling to breathe, their eyes filled with fear, were impossible to forget. But these moments also deepened my resolve to fight for every life, no matter the odds.

Through the Lens of a Pakistan-Based Physician-Scientist— Qalab Abbas

As COVID-19 hit the world, Pakistan—neighbouring China and Iran—was among the first few countries to be affected. Due to various reasons, such as scarce testing availability, limited reporting, and the stigma associated with the disease, not many cases were reported after the confirmation of the first case on February 26, 2020.

Pediatric intensive care in Pakistan is limited to a few major hospitals in some large cities of the country. Aga Khan University Hospital in Karachi is one of the largest private sector hospitals in the country, with a well-established pediatric intensive care unit, running on full capacity throughout the year. During the COVID-19 pandemic, it was commonly believed that children were mostly unaffected by severe symptoms, which offered us some reassurance. Nevertheless, many children with respiratory illnesses were tested, and strict precautions were enforced. Adjusting to this new reality was both difficult and time-consuming.

Dealing with Uncertainty

While we were dealing with COVID-19 and settling into the new "normal" within our broader community, we received few COVID-19-positive children. Some of them had co-infections, and the majority had comorbid conditions. There were many unanswered questions and a lot of uncertainty, which, although not unusual in the pediatric intensive care unit (PICU) in ordinary circumstances, was exaggerated in the context of the COVID-19 pandemic, for example, the uncertainty of whether to test once or repeatedly for COVID-19; which treatment to provide; and the effects of other infections and comorbidities on the manifestation of COVID-19 itself. In the initial days, we managed COVID-19 in children with supportive care and antibiotics, unsure of what would work and what would not. With so much news and literature coming from all over the world, keeping up with evidence base practices was exhausting. Our colleagues from infectious diseases took the lead and developed local and national guidelines for the management of COVID-19 in children, which provided clarity and some certainty.

The Professional Challenges

Professionally I witnessed helplessness, hopelessness, and resilience. Sometimes we were refusing patients (adults) due to unavailability of space, and I remember very vividly how sometimes we bypassed certain policies to get our own colleagues admitted. I even stayed with a colleague while he was admitted to the hospital.

During the first peak of COVID-19 pandemic, working as PICU doctor was a constant struggle against uncertainty, resource constraints, and ever-changing policies. Government policies fluctuated, driven by local and international emerging recommendations, with varied implementations across hospitals. Some larger hospitals had better compliance to guidelines for COVID-19 testing and management, while others were left to navigate the crisis with limited guidance and resources. Isolation rooms were scarce, and mostly, regular patient areas were converted to makeshift isolation units; proper masks (like N-95) were in short supply, being used without fit-testing; and alternatives were rarely available. Families, fearing stigma and overwhelmed hospitals, often brought children too late for timely management. There was also a lot of misinformation in the electronic and digital media, and it would take a long time for us to discuss and explain to the families the condition and what needed to be done for the best interest of the child. On discharge, parents would sometimes request that there be no mention of COVID-19 as a diagnosis on the discharge summaries. Being a PICU physician, it was very busy at some large tertiary care centres like ours, while others in smaller hospitals or those primarily working in cardiac ICU had significantly decreased burden, which also resulted in lesser revenue and pay cuts.

While we were settling in to manage the diagnosis of COVID-19, the presence of a new syndrome called "Multisystem Inflammatory Syndrome" (MIS) came to us. It affected children (MIS-C) more than adults (MIS-A) and those with more severe disease. We were unsure in the first few suspected cases about the definition and management of the syndrome. We worked alongside our cardiology colleagues in a group including experts from across the city and country as well as the World Health Organization (WHO) to define the syndrome. Subsequently, there was still uncertainty on many occasions about who to label MIS-C—some had comorbidity; some had infections—and there was always debate on whether to administer intravenous immunoglobulin (IVIg) or steroids.

As our load within the PICU increased, we commissioned a new PICU, on another floor, with less-than-optimal human and other resources—it opened among uncertainties and many unanswered questions about the management of COVID-19 patients. Despite this, the initiative was successful and offered services and care to more children. It was a treat and a reward to witness the team members coming forward to help and support each other during those testing times.

The Capacity for Research, Collaboration, and Global Outreach

The WHO Department of Maternal and Child Health invited me to be part of the newly formed MIS-C working group. We then met every other week to share experiences and management practices of COVID-19 in children generally and with MIS-C specifically. We developed a revised definition of MIS-C. At the end of the first year of the pandemic, the WHO convened a group of multidisciplinary physicians from across the world, to conduct a systematic review of MIS-C and present findings to the WHO guideline development group.

As we were settling into this uncertainty, along with treating critically ill children, I also led a WHO-funded study on severe COVID-19 in children across four countries including Pakistan. This research was conducted amidst extremely strained resources and stigma, revealing an alarming morbidity and mortality rates specially in Pakistan. More importantly, it reshaped bedside care, guiding treatment strategies, and fostering real-time exchange by sharing experiences across the borders, followed by local webinars. The data coming out of this also convinced the government to start vaccination for younger children.

The pandemic also redefined our role as PICU physicians. Beyond providing care at the bedside, I saw an unprecedented enthusiasm for collaboration and cross-learning. This also led to the rapid development and deployment of a tele-ICU platform that connected intensivists across hospitals in the country. For some remote and less resourced hospitals, these connections became a lifeline, allowing real-time discussion on case management, sharing the evolving protocols and co-learning. Later, enquiries related more to MIS-C, which increased our knowledge about the limitations and challenges our colleagues faced working in a resource-constrained environment. It was an enormous learning experience for me and my team. Later during the pandemic, I had the opportunity to visit some of these facilities and witness the care being provided firsthand to children, who make up one-third of the total population of Pakistan. Our team was subsequently able to evaluate the resources for provision of critical care across the country. For many of us, this pandemic was a defining moment in our careers, contributing to not only our own patients' care but also to a larger national and regional effort reinforced why we chose this field—to make an impact in times of crisis. I personally learnt to be adaptable to rapidly changing scenarios and to collaborate on a larger scale. The pandemic served to inspire doctors to strive to not underestimate our capacities but instead to work to make a larger impact not only as doctors but as leaders and innovators as well.

The Personal Highs and Lows in a Developing Nation

During the pandemic, as I finished work and headed home, the next thing on my mind was my own family, and thoughts of protecting them were enormously stressful. I made a separate area where I kept my shoes and scrubs, and I adopted a routine practice of showering before meeting them.

This time was also a reminder of the vulnerability that comes with being a PICU physician. Every day, we walked into the PICU knowing we were at risk, not just from virus itself but from the emotional toll of constant uncertainty. The fear of exposure was double, not only for our own self but our families back home. However, this did not deter us from why we chose PICU careers, a responsibility that defines the very essence of critical care for the most vulnerable.

Later during the pandemic, as restrictions eased, I was fortunate enough to travel to Iraq with a group of colleagues for a congenital heart disease mission in Najaf. This was beyond exciting for me, not only to see the healthcare infrastructure and care provision in war-torn countries but also for spiritual and religious reasons. Visiting the shrines of Ali and Hussain strengthened my bond with knowledge, curiosity, and humanity, sacrifice, and resilience. We have been going there regularly, and it gives me satisfaction and happiness to see that the PICU and congenital heart surgery program at Najaf is growing nicely, led now by their local teams.

What I Learned and Will Take Forward

I learned the importance of family presence with their dear ones during this pandemic more than any time before or after. During the early pandemic days, an 18-year-old boy with trisomy 21 was admitted to our hospital with COVID-19, and he had underlying severe pulmonary hypertension. As per standard precautions, his family was not allowed to visit him, and his condition continued to deteriorate. Since he was being looked after by the pediatric service before turning 18, he was known to us. The family approached us, and after many debates and necessary approvals for change of services from adult to pediatrics, he was shifted to our PICU, and we allowed his family members (who had recovered from COVID-19) to be with him. I saw how happy he was and how grateful the family was; he started improving, and we were able to discharge him home on BIPAP.

Emerging from the Pandemic and Moving Forward as Intensivists

What can the intensivists of tomorrow take away from the experiences of COVID-19 to prepare for the pandemics of the future?

1. The power of international collaboration: The pandemic underscored the importance of global cooperation in medicine. Early in the crisis, intensivists worldwide shared observations, treatment protocols, and data in real time, bridging gaps between resource-rich and resource-limited settings [1]. Virtual platforms connected healthcare professionals across continents, allowing for rapid knowledge exchange and implementation of best practices.

   • Collaborative efforts led to accelerated research, informing treatment strategies such as steroid use, proning techniques, and ventilator management.
   • International partnerships provided critical support to healthcare systems facing resource shortages, from ventilators to personal protective equipment.
   • The collective approach to clinical trials, including the RECOVERY and REMAP-CAP studies [2, 3], demonstrated that large-scale, multi-national research could generate robust, lifesaving evidence in record time.

   • For future intensivists, the lesson is clear: medicine is not confined by borders. The ability to communicate, collaborate, and adapt knowledge from global colleagues is essential for navigating the next pandemic.

2. The power of communication: Effective communication was one of the most powerful tools in managing the crisis. The ability to convey clear, science-backed information to colleagues, policymakers, and the public had a direct impact on outcomes.

   • Within hospitals, transparent and timely communication between leadership and frontline workers helped streamline workflows and adapt to rapidly changing guidelines.
   • Public health messaging played a critical role in shaping preventive measures, with some campaigns—such as the widely shared "Remy Effect" video [4]—directly influencing behaviour and policy.
   • Communicating with patients and families became an essential skill, particularly when visitor restrictions forced intensivists to become the only human connection for dying patients. The ability to provide compassionate, clear updates over a telephone became just as critical as clinical expertise.

   • Future intensivists must recognize that their role extends beyond clinical management; they are also educators, advocates, and, at times, the sole voice of comfort for families facing unimaginable loss.

3. The risk of miscommunication: Just as communication saved lives, miscommunication—intentional or unintentional—cost many. The pandemic highlighted how misinformation and public distrust can exacerbate crises.

   1. Conflicting guidelines from health organizations created confusion among both healthcare professionals and the public.
   2. The rapid spread of misinformation on social media fueled vaccine hesitancy, mask resistance, and denialism, leading to preventable deaths.
   3. The politicization of science eroded trust in experts, making it difficult for intensivists to implement necessary interventions without facing public backlash.

      For future pandemics, intensivists must be proactive in combatting misinformation. This includes engaging with public education, advocating for transparency in policy decisions, and ensuring that critical health messages are not diluted by political or media distortions.

4. Public perception of intensive care and intensive care doctors: The pandemic brought intensivists into the spotlight, altering public perception of what it means to be a critical care physician.

   - At the peak of the crisis, ICU doctors were hailed as heroes, their relentless efforts recognized in a way rarely seen before. Yet, as fatigue set in and misinformation spread, some sectors of the public turned against them, questioning their motives, their treatments, and even their integrity.
   - The reality of ICU care—prolonged suffering, difficult ethical decisions, and frequent mortality—was starkly exposed. Families who once saw ICUs as places of last hope also witnessed the painful reality that not all could be saved.
   - Some intensivists found a renewed passion for their work, embracing the role of patient advocate and public health educator. Others, burned out and disillusioned, left the field entirely.

Moving forward, intensivists must actively shape their profession's public image. The field needs more advocates who can educate the public on what ICU care entails, dispel myths about life-sustaining treatments, and build trust before the next crisis emerges.

Conclusion

The COVID-19 pandemic was a defining moment in critical care medicine, revealing both our vulnerabilities and our strengths. The intensivists of tomorrow must take these lessons to heart, recognizing that their role extends far beyond the bedside. The future of intensive care will depend on a commitment to collaboration, clear and effective communication, vigilance against misinformation, and a renewed effort to shape public perception of the field.

For those who choose to stand in the ICU during the next pandemic, the challenge will be immense—but so will the opportunity to lead, to heal, and to shape the future of medicine. Even when a deadly virus strips away human connection, strive to restore humanity—both in your patients and in the world around you. In the end, on some days, that may be the most meaningful thing we can offer.

References

1. Remy KE, Verhoef PA, Malone JR, Ruppe MD, Kaselitz TB, Lodeserto F, Hirshberg EL, Slonim A, Dezfulian C. Caring for critically ill adults with coronavirus disease 2019 in a PICU: recommendations by dual trained intensivists. Pediatr Crit Care Med 2020 J21(7):607–619. doi:https://doi.org/10.1097/PCC.0000000000002429. PMID: 32420720; PMCID: PMC7331597.
2. RECOVERY Collaborative Group, Horby P, Lim WS, Emberson JR, Mafham M, Bell JL, Linsell L, Staplin N, Brightling C, Ustianowski A, Elmahi E, Prudon B, Green C, Felton T, Chadwick D, Rege K, Fegan C, Chappell LC, Faust SN, Jaki T, Jeffery K, Montgomery A, Rowan K, Juszczak E, Baillie JK, Haynes R, Landray MJ. Dexamethasone in hospitalized patients with Covid-19. N Engl J Med. 2021;384(8):693–704. https://doi.org/10.1056/NEJMoa2021436. Epub 2020 Jul 17. PMID: 32678530; PMCID: PMC7383595
3. Angus DC, Berry S, Lewis RJ, Al-Beidh F, Arabi Y, van Bentum-Puijk W, Bhimani Z, Bonten M, Broglio K, Brunkhorst F, Cheng AC, Chiche JD, De Jong M, Detry M, Goossens H, Gordon A, Green C, Higgins AM, Hullegie SJ, Kruger P, Lamontagne F, Litton E, Marshall J, McGlothlin A, McGuinness S, Mouncey P, Murthy S, Nichol A, O'Neill GK, Parke R, Parker J, Rohde G, Rowan K, Turner A, Young P, Derde L, McArthur C, Webb SA. The REMAP-CAP (Randomized Embedded Multifactorial Adaptive Platform for Community-acquired Pneumonia) Study. Rationale and design. Ann Am Thorac Soc. 2020;17(7):879–91. https://doi.org/10.1513/AnnalsATS.202003-192SD. PMID: 32267771; PMCID: PMC7328186
4. https://youtu.be/PBwBeH-J0i4?si=fCZUyEtjEgzuYm0k

Part III
Learning to Sing

Foreword: How to Perform a Song

Denise Goodman

> Tell me and I forget, teach me and I may remember, involve me and I learn. (Benjamin Franklin)

Think of your favourite song or your favourite musical performance. It's clear that the artist has mastery of their instrument or voice. They've practiced with the other musicians; they know the lyrics, the chord changes, the nuts-and-bolts of music; then when all that is internalized, they channel it through their own experience; and they inhabit the music and make something new and beautiful.

You too can make something beautiful. You learn physiology and medications and the natural history of a condition. Then you fully become part of the moment and let all of these come together in the unique situation of that patient. It's the same not only with the clinical delivery of care but with your relationships with the patient, the family, the team and the whole hospital ecosystem. The following four chapters explore how you can metaphorically learn to "sing" as an intensivist.

It begins with learning the words—what is the other person saying, and then what are they really saying? In the George and Ira Gershwin song "They Can't Take That Away From Me", the lyrics start, "The way you wear your hat/The way you sip your tea/The memory of all that/No, no, they can't take that away from me". Are they singing about fashion or beverages? Of course not, they are singing about the fond memories of relationships. In the same way, we'll see how one really needs to listen deeply to hear the meaning behind the words that are used and needs to reflect carefully to choose one's own words. Then, how do you avoid cacophony? How do you take these disparate views and words and styles and make them harmonious? We'll see how you can balance these many voices and viewpoints. We'll also see how the unique situation of a critically ill child introduces its own challenges.

When it all comes together, it is like an orchestra, diverse in instrumentation but creating a complex, full sound pulling you in and moving as one from one section of music to another. It's like a choir, each voice unique, each person drawn to the song for his or her own reasons but joined as one into something far greater than any individual performance. A study of Swedish 18-year-olds singing as a choir showed that not only were their voices joined, but their heartbeats became synchronized [1]. There are moments in the ICU just like this, and it can become something to aspire to in our every interaction. Your experiences, your reflection, your self-awareness and your listening are all part of this song.

Reference

1. Bickhoff B, Malmgren H, Astrom R, et al. Music structure determines heart rate variability of singers. Front Psychol 2013 Jul 9;4:334. https://doi.org/10.3389/fpsyg.2013.00334. PMID 23847555

Chapter 11
Singing from the Same Songbook: Contemplating Communicating with Family

Mary Pinder

The difference between the right word and the almost right word is the difference between lightning and a lightning bug.

– *Mark Twain*

Communicating with the family members of patients is a key role for the intensive care clinician and can be very challenging but also very rewarding. Family members are themselves under stress and may display any or all of the range of emotions associated with grief and loss. Family members may also feel that they have lost control. There may also be a sense that the healthcare system has failed their loved one. These emotional responses may be expressed as anger and frustration and even aggression towards the healthcare team. Every family experiences instances of disharmony, and the stress of a having a family member critically ill in the ICU adversely affects family dynamics and can heighten any conflict.

Conversations with family members are stressful for the healthcare team. Knowing the words to use is so important, as they are integral to building trust, showing empathy, and providing information and emotional support. Members of the healthcare team are often in the position of communicating devastating news to family members when the patient has died or is not expected to survive and must manage their own emotional response to the loss of their patient.

We have already established that the ICU is a high-risk environment (Chap. 8), and adverse medical events are sadly inevitable. In general, adverse events reflect organisational issues rather than being the fault of an individual. However, healthcare workers must deal with their own feelings of guilt, self-blame, and anxiety and at the same time communicate honestly and openly with the family to explain the course of events and expected outcomes. The ICU healthcare team must also manage conflict with members of other healthcare teams involved in patient care, and

M. Pinder (✉)
Department of Intensive Care, Sir Charles Gairdner Hospital, Perth, Australia
e-mail: mary.pinder@health.wa.gov.au

© The Author(s), under exclusive license to Springer Nature Switzerland AG 2025
D. Dennis et al. (eds.), *Contemplating the Role of an Intensive Care Doctor*,
https://doi.org/10.1007/978-3-031-92766-9_11

this is also a source of stress—discussed more in Chap. 12. In all of this, the ICU clinician must resolve differences of opinion and remain an advocate for the patient to ensure the best outcome and ensue that the family does not lose trust in the healthcare team.

Family members may come from a background of diverse cultural, spiritual, and personal beliefs and values that may influence their interaction with the healthcare team. There may be requests for non-standard interventions that may have no impact on overall patient care and in some instances may be potentially harmful. The intensive care clinician must negotiate the challenge of refusing requests for inappropriate therapies while showing respect for the family's beliefs and maintaining their confidence and trust in the healthcare team. The following quotations illustrate some of the challenges relating to communication with families and provide a platform for reflection and discussion.

Family Dynamics

My experience in dealing with families in adverse events is both enriching, and inspiring, and immensely frustrating, and it depends on the family. I think you have extraordinarily caring and nurturing and reasonable families that you admire and deal with. And you think, "Wow, this was a bunch of really united people caring for each other, and work as a unit, and care about the patient, and want the best, and understand the difficulties of what we do". Or, you have a dysfunctional family, well beyond whatever it is that you do or say, they are already in full- blown intra-family conflict, where an adverse event then becomes actually a tool for enlarged and more aggressive intra-family conflict.

- While supporting families who come together during a crisis of illness can teach us humility and understanding, those families already experiencing conflict can fall further apart. Sometimes there is scope for the intensivist to help families navigate the tensions; sometimes the intensivist will find themselves at the centre of tensions. Two extremes of family dynamics are described in this quote. Reflecting on any experience you have had with either or both types of family dynamic, what was the context and what factors do you think had resulted in this dynamic?
- What steps would you take in preparing for a conversation with a family in whom tensions and conflict have been identified?
- How might tension/conflict be demonstrated during the family conversation?
- What strategies could you use at the start of and during the conversation to mitigate tension/conflict?
- How would you measure the outcome of the conversation in terms of achieving sharing of information?
- What might be the barriers to effective information sharing, and how would you mitigate each of these?

- What might be the benefits, and what might be the pitfalls in communicating with families in whom there is no apparent conflict or tension?
- How might family dynamics influence our care of the patient and their family member?

Establishing Trust

I think you have to always realise that unless the family is harming their [family member], it's generally an alliance, and if they don't trust you, it doesn't really matter what you do, it's not going to work well.

- What can contribute to patients and families not having trust with the healthcare team?
- What have you done in the past to build trust with your patients and their families outside the ICU setting? How have you maintained trust once this has been established?
- How can we build trust with patients and families in ICU?
- What are the barriers to building trust in the ICU setting, and what can be done to mitigate them?
- Sometimes a family will have trust in some members or groups within the healthcare team but not others. Reflecting on such a situation, consider who were the trusted members or groups, and who were those who weren't trusted and how this came to be. What might have been done differently to prevent or minimise loss of trust? How could, or how was, trust rebuilt?
- What are the consequences of a lack of trust to the patient, their family, and the healthcare team?

Losing Trust

An elderly man who had undergone a pancreatectomy a few days before, was due to be discharged to the ward that morning. As the nurse entered the room the patient was witnessed to have a large vomit. She suctioned the mouth and airway and called for help immediately, but the patient arrested and did not respond to multiple rounds of CPR and died. The family was advised and a few days later asked for an appointment to discuss the circumstances of the death. It was very clear from the outset of the discussion that they were very suspicious of anything I said. This became even more so when they asked to see the video of the event (all the ICU rooms have cameras recording all the time) and were told that the video was on a loop and new events had been recorded over the time when their father had died.

- How do you approach a conversation with a family where, clearly, they have lost trust in the medical team?
- When do you think is the best time to have this conversation with the family? Allow them time to grieve, and then speak to them or address their concerns as soon as possible?
- What would your response be if they indicated that they wished to record the conversation? What if you discovered that they were recording the conversation surreptitiously—how would you feel and how would you react?
- In a difficult meeting such as this, what would be the pros and cons of asking other professionals such as the head nurse and/or the unit social worker to also be present? How do you think this would be viewed by the family?
- How would you go about documenting the family discussion? What would lead you to report or not to the hospital legal team/risk management team?
- How would you end the discussion—for example, would you invite the family to a further discussion should they wish; would you forcefully end the discussion if they are aggressive?
- How would you personally decompress after such a difficult and potentially contentious conversation?

Supporting the Family Through the Dying Process

You want to keep going and not give up, but then, you realise that the writing's on the wall, so how do you transition the care to not escalating; to comfort; or let the parents hold the child; try to make the… It's not the right thing to say, to make it less traumatic, but try to give them… a path as smooth as it can be?

I focus my energy on building good rapport with the family, so that I can help them through that horrible process…. Trying to prepare that family; build rapport; demonstrating to them that I'm doing everything I can for their child; and helping them to see that even with all of the things that we are doing for them, it may not be enough. And so, in that way we can sort of… You know it's such a privilege of our jobs to walk a family through the death of their child.

- Helping a patient and their family make the transition from hope of recovery to acceptance of death is an important role of the intensivist. Reflect on your experience of this, whether it is something you have facilitated yourself or witnessed or maybe just thought about.
- This role carries a big responsibility, and the author of the quote describes seeing it as a privilege. How do you feel about taking on this role?
- If you have witnessed or played an active part in this situation, what was the context—was it a natural progression of care, or was it unexpected? What did you learn from this experience?
- What steps might you, or did you, take to prepare yourself for this role?

- What might be the barriers to doing this role well, and how you might anticipate and overcome these?
- What might be the positive aspects of this role?
- Supporting patients and families through the dying process can be very stressful. What strategies do you use to help you cope with stress? How can you recognise and help your team members who are experiencing stress?

Sharing Devastating News

You almost start your grieving process for that child before they even arrive. So, we hear about a kid who has had a full arrest from asthma, let's say. And they had an initial pH of 6.5; then they had 45 minutes of CPR; and 15 rounds of epi... before they even get to the hospital, for hours before... I know, okay this child is going to die there's nothing I can do to save them; I'm going to transition my focus to the family and try to really focus on being direct and clear with them, but also not being cruel and being honest; and if I can do that in a way that by the end, they say "thank you so much for your care, it really meant a lot", to me, that is a success.

- In this situation, the author of the quote knew from the outset that the prognosis for the patient was poor and had no pre-existing relationship with the family. If you were in a similar situation, what would be your mindset when meeting the family for the first time?
- What steps would you take to prepare yourself for the meeting, and what information would you like to have beforehand?
- What would be your framework for this conversation? How much information would you give?
- Who should be present at this meeting?
- How can you build rapport with the family in this situation?
- How can you check the family's understanding of your message?
- What follow-up will you arrange at the conclusion of this meeting?
- Sharing devastating news, such as of a sudden and unexpected death, is traumatic, especially with family you have not previously met. What strategies do you, or would you, use to help debrief and de-stress in this situation?

Navigating the Spectrum of Acceptance

We had a patient where one parent did not accept that the patient had a devastating neurologic injury. And she countered (anything we said) with, "When you're not in the room, he talks to me; he sits up" ... and he didn't even breathe on the ventilator... And so that was a very hard situation to deal with... I knew

that no matter what I said or what I knew, her reality was different. I've had families who have had this kind of… denial before, and if you keep pushing them, they respond with anger and mistrust. And sometimes aggression, and sometimes acting out. But you know…there's no way that I could put my truth into her.

We went and saw him; pupils fixed and dilated; we had to intubate and all that; scanned him; he had two huge frontal lesions… The kid was brain-dead from the time we met him. They refused to accept that.

There are families where clearly things haven't gone well. Patients were going well before, and they're dead now. And they've just still thanked the team for what they've done, and that can almost be as hard, because we want, as humans, to convey how sorry we are, or that we don't feel like we did our best, and the family are being, almost too nice about it.

- Within the context of ICU, every family has different dynamics, responses, and coping strategies when it comes to an acute medical situation involving their loved one. Reflect on this diversity of responses that you have seen so far in your medical career, and think of some of the more extreme reactions. How did you manage your own response and what did you learn?
- If the family are not accepting of an expected poor outcome, what effect does this have on your interactions with the patient and family?
- What strategies might help facilitate the family's acceptance of the outcome?
- What pressure do you think that places on the healthcare team?
- What are the positive and negative aspects of the situation where the family are apparently very accepting of the outcome?
- If a family meet you and your team with acceptance and grace when you feel you might have 'done better', how would you respond to them, and how do you imagine you would feel?
- Cultural and spiritual beliefs may be a factor in a family's level of acceptance. Reflect on how your own beliefs may influence your communication with families.

Family Requesting Appropriate Interventions

I (have) realised that maybe we shouldn't be so rigid about what we do, and if the family says, "Hey in the past, every time she's done this, the only thing that helped her was this…" I would say, "Alright well let me try it. I'm concerned about this and if this happens here's how we going to try to alleviate that, but if you still want to go ahead, let's give it a shot".

- Reflect on a situation where you and/or the healthcare team have been challenged about the management decisions for the patient. How did this make you feel? What was the outcome—was treatment changed? How did this affect ongoing interaction with the patient and family?

- How would you rebuild trust in this situation if that had been compromised?
- What do you think are the important aspects of the conversation with a family requesting specific and appropriate interventions for their family member?
- Families of patients with chronic conditions are often very well informed about the condition in question and the needs of their family member. How comfortable do you feel in being able to admit to your lack of knowledge or experience?
- Families may request interventions with no risk of harm but that align with their cultural, spiritual, and personal beliefs. How can you facilitate their request?

Family Requesting Inappropriate Interventions

There was another patient who was clearly dying… who the family … demanded all sorts of really unusual treatments, like … crystals… we'd never heard of this, so I was elected to go and talk to them, I think. So, I sat down with the whole family, and they told me how they had been recommended by this doctor to give [trademark of crystals], and why weren't we doing it? I went away and looked it up on the Internet and found that it was [a substance] which had been banned by the TGA. When I looked up the doctors they had recommended [it], they were doctors of letters not Doctor of Medicine ... I went back to them, and I said, "I've looked into this, and I'm sorry we can't give it, the TGA has actually banned it, and I explained what that meant, and I said it's actually likely to hasten the death of your family member".

- What do you think may motivate families to request interventions that are deemed inappropriate?
- If the family of one of your patients requested an intervention that you considered would be of no benefit, but no harm, to the patient, how would you deal with the situation?
- If the family of one of your patients requested an intervention that you considered to be potentially harmful, how would you deal with the situation?
- How might requests from the family for inappropriate interventions affect the relationship between the family and the healthcare team?
- How can you mitigate any adverse impact on the family-healthcare relationship that might occur as a consequence of refusing requests for interventions deemed inappropriate?

Explaining Multi-disciplinary Management Decisions

Where the surgeons are dragging their feet and don't want to go back, and we have to resuscitate, and resuscitate and eventually they take them back. In those cases, I do usually present the surgeon's side—that they are hoping that

this bleeding is going to stop, and we're going to do everything we can to avoid going back to the operating room, but if that's ultimately what's needed then that will happen. So, leaving open that possibility such that the family isn't in the middle… I try not to make the family a part of those conversations… or to make it worse. To say, "I really think that they need to go back to the operating room, but the surgeon won't take them"—I don't think that that would be useful. And so I think that my stance is always to try to say, "These are all things were going to do right now and if they aren't working, we will need to talk to the surgeons…" or "Just so you know, we're talking to the surgeons every hour and telling them what we're doing", so that the family knows that we are doing everything that we can, and that ultimately, it's up to the surgeon, but that we are advocating for their child. But I try not to make it an "us versus them" thing. We are all trying to figure out what's best.

- Reflect on a situation you have experienced where there has been conflict or disagreement about patient management between healthcare teams involved in that patient's care. What was the context and what was the outcome?
- What are factors that may lead to conflict or disagreement between healthcare teams?
- What might be the effect of conflict or disagreement on patient outcome?
- How can you do to maintain open and honest communication and trust with the family when there is conflict or disagreement between healthcare teams?
- What characteristics of diplomacy and negotiation might you demonstrate in communication with the family?
- In a situation like the one described, how do you navigate a three-way shared understanding of the situation and available options?

Coping with Grief

The mother is standing there screaming, "You killed my child" the whole time we were resuscitating the child. She ended up like, screaming for an hour straight; and so it's just… The child unfortunately was going to die; regardless of the intervention; but as a mother, I might have done the same thing, right? You just don't know in that situation. When you are facing so much grief; and while I realised it wasn't a personal attack, for her, I was the face of the death of her child.

So, the family walks in, and the mother starts crying. And she looks at me and she says, "Every time… I'm sorry but every time I see your face I think of my dead child" because I was the one… (there).

- This is one of the very confronting roles of any leader within medicine. When the patient dies, you may be seen by the family as the face of the healthcare team, and, as an extension of that, sometimes the 'face of death'. What might you and the healthcare team do to support the family in their grief?

- What communication strategies can you use to acknowledge the family's grief?
- What are some of the different ways family members might show grief?
- Reflect on how you are affected by a patient's death. How do your own emotions influence your interaction with the family?
- How does your response to one patient's death and interaction with their family affect your interaction with other patients and other families?
- What coping strategies do you use to help you recover from a patient's death?

Avoiding Blame and Speculation in Open Disclosure

I actually try very hard to not try to explain care that I was not part of… learn to talk about what you know. And it's hard to know when you are not part of the experience. So, I try really hard not to engage in speculation or trying to figure out what happened from the standpoint of like an error or something beforehand… Because I've had families who ask, "So did they do the wrong thing"? or "Did they make a mistake"? And I always try not to deflect, but to explain to the family that is very hard to know when you're not part of the situation, exactly what transpired and that what's important right now is to focus on "This is what we know is going on right now", and "These are the things that we need to do to try to understand what's happening with your child, treat your child or whatever…" wherever we are at in that trajectory. To say that it's understandable that there are questions that they have, but that we are not the best people to answer them, like our team, if we weren't involved in that… care. And try to maintain the focus on here and now.

I'm very careful not to blame other doctors because I didn't see them; I wasn't there; they had a lack of situational awareness—as all humans do—as to what else was going on; you know?

- ICU is a high-risk environment, and open disclosure with communication of regret is crucial in the event of medical error. What are the benefits of open disclosure to the patient, family, healthcare team, and healthcare system?
- During open disclosure it is important to be truthful and factual and avoid speculation when there is genuine uncertainty around the course of events and to avoid apportioning blame when there are faults with the system as a whole. How do the quotes listed here support this statement?
- What steps can be taken to ensure optimal timing of open disclosure?
- What steps can be taken to ensure that the communication is not perceived to apportion blame?
- Guilt and self-blame are common emotional responses for healthcare workers involved in an instance of medical error. Reflect on what your response may be in this situation. What coping strategies are available to help process this emotional response? How would you seek support to help you?

Coping with Threatening Behaviours

One of the nurses said, "Hey, the family is threatening to hurt you" I was pregnant at the time... "To hurt your baby"... I didn't think they were serious... But it was enough that... it was one where I sort of looked over my shoulder a little bit....

We had a family say that they would bring a gun in and shoot us if their child died. That was not a good environment to work in.

I've had families get very physically threatening, like up in my face. Yelling, "You need to fix this…" You know when things aren't going well; or things are just the way they are, it's not like the kid is arresting or acutely dying right there, but they're not getting better the way the family wants them to get better so there's anger. And sometimes it's about communication issues. They heard one thing from one team, and they get frustrated. And some families don't have the coping skills, but others do, and they are yelling and threatening to…

I did have a mother call, after her child died, and say, "That probably, if I knew what was good for me, I should leave town and not live in..." you know... she didn't want me to be practicing medicine here anymore; and that maybe I should…

We have had patient's families in the unit who have been abusive and that has become very tense in the unit. We have had to involve the police or security in the unit to try to protect the staff.

I start by giving families as much grace as possible, whether that equates to giving them more time to process difficult news or more latitude to lash out or question everything. That's not to say it's OK to tolerate being verbally abused, but it's easy to forget how foreign an ICU is for most people. Regardless of their "day job", this is likely a terrifying situation and few people are prepared to know how to act.

I try to pause and consider how I might act if I were the scared, grieving family member and the tables were turned. Would I be able to remain polite if the ICU doctor told me they didn't know exactly what was wrong and didn't know if my loved one was going to live? I doubt that uncertainty and stress would be easy to handle. To expect families to use manners and be reasonable every day is not reasonable. That is perpetually the condition that we are asking our patient's families to exist in.

- What might be the factors leading to a family member displaying threatening behaviour?
- What strategies might you use to de-escalate aggressive or threatening behaviour in a family conversation?
- How would you seek advice and support within your organisation related to receiving threats from any source?

- How can you minimise the risk of exposure to threatening behaviour from family members?
- How can you support team members who have been exposed to threatening behaviour?
- Reflect on how you would feel if 'the tables were turned' and you were a family member of a patient in ICU. How do you think you would act in this situation?

Conclusion

Communicating with the families of our patients is an integral part of our job as part of the ICU healthcare team. This is an opportunity to build rapport and trust and can be hugely rewarding and at times challenging and stressful. Family members' reactions can be very confronting, and we should remember that, unlike us, they do not get to hand over to a colleague and go home at the end of their shift. It is important to remember that, however senior we are, we are not going to get it right every time and we will make mistakes. We need to be kind to ourselves, foster coping strategies, build resilience, and develop our communication skills through workshops, courses, and discussion with colleagues and mentors.

Chapter 12
Melodies and Harmonies: Contemplating Communicating with Other Doctors

Michael Ruppe (iD)

> *No one can whistle a symphony. It takes a whole orchestra to play it.*
>
> *– H.E. Luccock*

The ICU doctor, simply by the nature of their craft, is subject to preconceived assumptions. They can be seen as hubris-filled adrenaline junkies and not balanced, sensible colleagues. This makes communication with other doctors uniquely challenging and often imbalanced, to the detriment of patient care. This chapter describes how ICU doctors may run the risk of being unrelatable, as they gravitate towards the extreme end of illness severity and can exude a blasé attitude about the remaining features of a complex patient, particularly when a patient is being considered for ICU admission and the referring doctor may feel like their story needs to be a sales pitch to woo the ICU gatekeeper. To facilitate best patient-centred care, ICU doctors should seek to sing somewhat of the same melody as their colleagues from other teams, in a joined harmony.

Communication challenges between doctors can take many forms such as hierarchical power struggles, imbalances in perception or experience, and even outright disagreements about the 'right' course of action. These moments can degrade into personality clashes and can severely impact medical decision-making at a crucial time. Lasting damage to personal and professional relationships between doctors is often at stake. The quotations throughout this section illustrate these scenarios and are paired with questions for ICU doctors to become as prepared to navigate these challenges as possible.

When responding to urgent situations throughout the hospital, the ICU doctor needs to pause and 'read the room'. This can be 'tiptoeing' into shared management in the context of sick patient in an emergency room trauma bay or 'diving in

M. Ruppe (✉)
University of Louisville Department of Pediatrics, Division of Critical Care,
and Norton Children's Medical Group, Louisville, KY, USA
e-mail: michael.ruppe@louisville.edu

D. Dennis et al. (eds.), *Contemplating the Role of an Intensive Care Doctor*,
https://doi.org/10.1007/978-3-031-92766-9_12

headfirst' into stabilizing a critical patient following a decompensation on the medical ward. The communication style needs to be as nuanced and customized as the location, patient condition, and provider type that they encounter. A fixed mindset of aggressive, tunnel vision towards ICU care will often be a disservice to optimal communication and interpersonal relationships. As previously explored, the ICU doctor may need to assume various personas (Chap. 6) and roles (Chap. 7) to fit the situation. Throughout this chapter, we provide examples of circumstances that demand this flexibility. We also provide questions that will allow introspection and hopefully arm and prepare ICU doctors to optimally communicate during these encounters.

Being Unimpressed by Acuity

I think the stereotype would be that we are very intense people; we may not be so approachable; we may be… we may sort of…downplay their… because we see the sickest ones… we may not be as "accepting"… Like when they have a sick kid, and they think that the child is sick and ill; we may look at it and say, "It's fine". We're hard to impress when it comes to the critical piece of the illness. And so, in that way, leading to that "not very approachable" piece. Like we will just "blow them off". But I think one of the things I've always said, and I always try to teach the Fellows too, is it doesn't matter how comfortable you are it's about how uncomfortable the other person is. If the other person is not comfortable taking care of the patient, the other person is not comfortable taking care of the patient, and they're asking for our help. Even though you think it's totally fine, yep…

- The key piece of this quote is that there needs to be a level of understanding and empathy towards doctors in other areas when they reach out for help, advice, or expertise. Rest assured; they too may not be comfortable being uncomfortable! How do you explicitly demonstrate respect to a colleague who is on the phone *or with you at the bedside*, asking you for advice regarding their patient?
- What are the barriers to effective consultation inherent within the context of a conversation?
- How important is it for you to demonstrate empathy?
- If the case does not meet the criteria for a transfer to your care, do you provide ongoing support to this colleague once the conversation ends, and if so, how do you do this?
- How do you decipher if the colleague is solely seeking advice or if what they are really asking is for a discussion about transfer to the ICU?
- How does this exchange lend itself to standardization and documentation in the medical record?

Handover Issues

When we handed off from the night team to the day team—I was part of the day team—and I don't think that handoff… I don't think we… we did not ask all of the clarifying questions that we needed to ask. And we just got a general, "She was doing okay", which could have meant a lot of different things… we probably didn't ask the right questions to elicit this (important additional) information, and neither did the night team offer it to us.

When someone receives a piece of knowledge and doesn't understand its impact, they may fail to communicate it… However, you didn't think to articulate that "If this happens, you need to tell me". You don't know what you don't know. But do I know what you don't know?

- Handoff or handover is a fundamental component of contemporary healthcare practice across all disciplines and all professions. The overall acuity and multifactorial nature of illness in the intensive care setting however make detailed, relevant, and succinct handover challenging. The specialty teams who are managing care change, and each may have different frames from which they view the patient. What may be important to one team is less important to another. Who decides which team's view should dictate? Treatment priorities change, with things that seemed important yesterday being less important today. The person at the centre of this, keeping all the balls in the air without them dropping is, of course, the intensivist. Have you reflected on how you do or will manage this oversight?
- Ongoing regular communication between medical specialty teams is key. In your experience, what barriers exist to this practice? How might you overcome these?
- Do you currently use any tools to facilitate better communication with other medical specialty teams?
- How do you mediate differing subspecialist recommendations when they oppose each other? For example, a pulmonologist may recommend additional diuresis to improve lung health, while a nephrologist may recommend administering additional fluid boluses to improve hydration and renal function.
- Think about a time when poor communication around patient care was evident between doctors from different medical specialty teams. What allowed the situation to evolve? Did it persist? What solutions were put in place to remediate the situation?
- What have you learned in your day-to-day practice to address the challenges of communicating handover?
- How can you minimize distortion of the clinical plans between day and night ICU teams? How can communication during handoff pre-empt problems with consistency?

Running a Resuscitation Outside of the ICU

I think it almost always should be the intensivist. The problem is, in an out-of-intensive-care-area, when you have a senior registrar and an emergency department (ED) consultant, I think in that scenario, probably the ED consultant is reasonable to run the resus; and then you've got generally a highly skilled ICU fairly advanced trainee who can assist with access and lines, and I think that's probably reasonable. I think in the case where there is an intensivist there, and you have left the ED, then an intensivist should run the resus… it's important for us to take ownership and responsibility for the situation when you walk into the room. You need to gather information fairly quickly and then announce to the room that you are going to lead. Obviously if it's an arrest you might be announcing that fairly quickly. If it's a just a sick patient, then you might have that time to take a hand over and then say, "Okay I might take over from you guys" and run it from there.

- 'Taking over' the lead of a medical emergency response is not always an easy thing to do, especially in unfamiliar circumstances and with unfamiliar people. Are you the most senior in the room? Are you the most qualified? Have you had to do this before? What are the realities of resuscitating patients in unfamiliar locations outside of the ICU?
- If you have, how did you know that it was the most appropriate role to assume, and how did you announce to the group that you were 'taking charge'?
- If you have not, how do you think you will navigate this?
- With limited overall knowledge of the patient's condition, how do you optimize the experience of the team that knows the patient the best while establishing your role in a leader capacity?
- Consider if there might be a situation where you would not take the lead role. What other role would you assume? Is designating yourself as a 'proceduralist' appropriate?
- If you decided not to take the lead role, is there a process whereby you would re-evaluate the role allocation within the team that was attending the event? What would that look like?

Conveying a Shared Understanding

There was not a recognition of the fact that her pain, which required escalating doses of narcotic medicine, was an indicator of something very bad. She was actually still stable in terms of her vital signs, but our Fellow recognised the situation, made recommendations; and then left the room, because the patient's vital signs were stable; expecting that until she was transferred to the ICU that the recommendations would be pursued… there wasn't a recognition of the

fact that this patient was really high risk by the staff that were left to care for her. So the recommendations were not pursued in an urgent fashion; and unfortunately by the time the Fellow returned to the bedside, the patient had decompensated, and was in completely uncompensated haemorrhagic shock, and was not able to be resuscitated. Our Fellow was really disappointed because she felt that she had conveyed the urgency of the situation, but it was not received in that way.

- Having a shared understanding of the acuity of any critical situation is important. What are the barriers to doctors from different specialties gaining this collective awareness?
- How do you ensure that another doctor appreciates the urgency of an instruction you relay?
- How do you think you would feel in a situation where, with hindsight, you feel you under-communicated the urgency of a situation and patient care was compromised?
- Overtly stated and direct communication is crucial when responding to critical patient needs in unfamiliar locations. Inferences and vague speech can have major implications. How do you frame a summary of a patient's condition that accurately reflects their condition and gives a clear and concise plan?

Understanding Another Team's Perspective

I feel like if I'm advocating for them to go back to the operating room for like a bleeding abdomen, I can generally see their (the surgeon's) side and why they are hoping that medical management will work. That it's not because they're lazy, it's not because they just don't want to go back; it's because they have a good reason, so I don't really…. I generally try to trust that they have good reasons to not go back, and I will do the best that I can with the tools that I have knowing that there are limitations as to what that can accomplish. And so, I think in those circumstances I tend to not get angry, I tend to be like constantly… It's very stressful, it is… But to be trying to understand their perspective…

- It is easy to become exasperated by a perceived lack of engagement from another team in terms of them agreeing with your perspective, and the classic scenario is whether an urgent return to theatre for a patient is needed or appropriate. This quote advocates for sensitivity and trust around the professional judgment of another specialty. Have you ever been in a situation or witnessed an incident where an intensivist was frustrated at the lack of engagement of another specialty in the care of a patient, but in the end the other team was seen to have provided appropriate and adequate oversight? How did it make you feel?
- What did you learn from the situation?

- What would you seek to do the next time that a scenario like this plays out for you?
- The adage 'if you're a hammer everything looks like a nail' can be applied to the varying mindsets of subspecialists caring for complex patients. Understanding this reality, how can you see through the eyes of other doctors and moderate the strategy that is best for the patient? Is that always a realistic possibility?

Not Understanding Another Team's Perspective

The kid was looking worse and worse; and the [other specialty] didn't want to come see her; and finally, my ICU Fellow had to say, "This patient needs to go to the operating room, they're coming to the intensive care unit" and the patient looked... for all intents and purposes, almost dead. Like she was yellow, and barely breathing, and the [other specialty] Fellow walked in, and wouldn't talk to our team... Next thing they know, the kids going to the operating room.

We had a patient who was decompensating in front of us, and we needed to go back to the OR for surgery, and the surgeons were actually on board to do it, but the anaesthesiologist came up and said, "They are too sick" and refused to take him. And that, I got really angry about. Because the reason they were so sick was that they needed surgery... The surgery was delayed for something like six hours and the child was that much worse... It was a very frustrating thing to be a part of.

- The flipside is when another specialty does not understand the urgent nature of the request by the intensivist to revisit a patient for whom they deem needs review. These quotes speak to a well-founded frustration on the part of the intensivist. Have you ever been in a situation or witnessed an incident where there was a lack of engagement from another specialty in the care of a patient and in the end the other team was found to have provided inadequate oversight? How did it make you feel?
- What did you learn from the situation?
- What would you seek to do the next time that a scenario like this plays out for you?
- Scenario 65 illustrates a path towards understanding both sides of a scenario, while the examples in scenario 66 show how incomplete information or delayed communication can be detrimental. When have you been upset with crucial communication breakdowns? What are ways to mitigate the injury?
- After communication breakdown with resultant patient harm, what constructive, prospective processes can you employ to prevent future harm?

Earning Trust

I think that the more they trust you, the more they share. You can see why they wouldn't necessarily dictate all of that in an operative note. You know, "There was a thousand things bleeding, we got control of 987 of those; we feel that at this point, this is the best option moving forward…" That's not something you're going to dictate, but in reality, that sometimes is the greyness of what they're dealing with…

- Sometimes there is a perception that surgeons do not openly share everything with the intensive care team, and this can feel disharmonious and counterproductive. After all, the patient should be at the centre of everything. From their perspective, they may be handing over everything they think is relevant rather than everything. Perhaps there is uncertainty as to whether things like bleeding are contained or not; perhaps they believe they have already done all that they could. The pragmatic solution is to maintain open lines of communication and not be afraid to voice concern if needed. How do you ensure that you receive all the information you need at handover to optimise a patient?
- Operations are often laborious and can take full days to complete. ICU handoffs from surgeons usually last less than 5 min. Given this disparity, how can an intensivist glean the reality of a complex surgery and know the crucial information to carry forward the recovery?
- What can an intensivist do to ensure the surgeons that their efforts in the theatre are understood and a clear plan, with contingency plans, is in place?
- When postoperative patients deteriorate, the dance between the surgeon and the intensivist can degrade into anger and blame. If this happens, what strategies can you use to refocus on restoring health yet fully address concerns from both sides?

The Grief of Other Specialties

We get [other specialties] who are very upset, and you can virtually see them go through the… it's the ABC of grieving. You know they're at the "denial" stage. They'll be at "angry" in two hours. You know, you can see it, so you need to have a really good understanding of other people.

- Sometimes doctors from other specialties have fought long and hard to maintain the health of a patient and avoid the need for ICU admission. This quote reflects an understanding of the commitment and investment that doctors can feel towards their patients that is developed over time following sustained periods of involvement in the management of their illness and adversity. Little wonder that they themselves may grieve the patient's admission to intensive care. Is this something you have considered?

- In hindsight, do you think you have ever experienced the stages of grief manifesting in doctors related to the status of their patient? Even if you have not, what do you imagine you might do to meet your colleague where they are at in that moment?
- When is it appropriate to console other specialists?
- What is the intensivist's emotional obligation (if any) to the colleague who has a long-standing relationship with a new ICU patient?

Denying Disagreement

I have felt anguish and conflict when you disagreed with a plan to begin with, and it was sort of forced upon you. Someone will make a decision, and the downstream (outcome) is bad, and you have to pick up the pieces. The next thing you know, they're doing a "revisionist history" in the sense that (they say), "I never said that"; "I never engaged in that behaviour"; or you know "I would never do it that way". And you think, well 12 hours ago you just did that, or said just that, or defended exactly the position you are now discarding...

- The intensivist is the master of managing the big picture and appreciating the long-term sequelae of decisions made upstream. Sometimes this is because they are the retrievers of patients for whom these decisions were made in the moment; sometimes it is because it is them who are the first to question an intervention where the outcome is identifiably futile. Having other doctors 'own' their decision-making seems to be an important piece of an intensivist maintaining their personal well-being. How might you ensure that ownership of decision-making is apportioned and transparent?
- If you encounter a situation where the 'revisionist history' described in the quote is evident, how do you think you will manage your feelings and practical response towards that doctor or that team?
- How do you think you might help your team to respond to the matter of 'revisionist history'?
- The flipside of this scenario is one in which you have made a decision that ultimately was deemed incorrect. This allows you to see the impact that incrimination or judgement can have. How can you depersonalize these realities in a way that preserves relationships while confronting the error directly?

Asking the Opinion of Other Specialties

I could think of 10 things that I wouldn't know how to handle or what to do with right now, but the likelihood of those coming in, is extremely rare and nobody else knows what to do with them either! And what we're gonna do is

we're gonna consult four different smart people and together the five of us will figure it out… And that sort of recognition, of, "Hey, we're in a system that has tons of really smart well-trained people", all I do, and this is the way I think about it now, is I'm the quarterback. My job is just to distribute to all these great players, and you don't have to do anything but integrate the information they're giving you and make a logical plan.

- An empowering sentiment is the acknowledgement of the team of people that surround the intensivist and share the burden of perceived omniscience. The quote permits a degree of ignorance and advocates for teamwork with the adage that 'many brains are better than one'. How does this sit with you?
- Is it appropriate to occasionally keep the patient 'alive', while the 'smarter' people figure out the problem?
- Think of a time when you found yourself in a position clinically where you had none of the answers and struggled to know which direction to take. How did it make you feel?
- How did you manage those feelings?
- How did those around you respond to you during this time?
- What did you learn from this situation?

Being Non-judgmental of Other Specialties

… for every person you see that things haven't gone right, there are maybe 90 or more that we never see because things *have* gone right. So, you have a selection bias, a real misperception of reality because you are in the cage. So be careful not to think that this surgeon doesn't know how to… (because) all you're seeing is the one that has gone wrong.

Part of coping with intensive care is acknowledging that people don't mean to fail. Systems don't mean to fail. They do, and we build in catchers to catch it, and that's *our* role. And our role is not to be persecutory to those that haven't lived up to the best standard. It is to support the patient and then support our colleagues as well.

You are going to be in unfortunate situations where, you come on and something else has happened or is presented to you after it has happened… As a profession, I think we should be trying to be less judgmental of others. I think ICUs are very much about "that surgeon did this"; "that person did that", "and now we've got to bail them out". And I don't think that that is a healthy long-term sort of attitude to take… It's difficult, but I have tried to be more aware of being just more accepting. My job is to be here to help whoever, and if I can… You need to be critical where it is appropriate but try to leave the value-based judgements at the door, and just accept and respond…

- It may be that the most brilliant surgeon agrees to consider and undertake the most difficult of cases because they offer the best chance of a successful outcome. On the receiving end of these sick post-operative patients however, the intensivist's perception may be that patients of this doctor are disproportionally represented in their intensive care case mix. Have you considered this selection bias?
- As an intensive care doctor, think about the important part you play in working with this brilliant surgeon. Do you think there is reciprocal understanding and acknowledgement of the role you both have in optimising the patient's condition?
- What prospective actions might you take to enhance this relationship?
- With the exception of those following standardised post-operative pathways, patients don't often arrive in ICU without some cascade of events that have climaxed in their high acuity. Sometimes it can be tempting to pass judgement on colleagues who appear to have contributed to that cascade either in what they have done or what they have failed to do as part of the patient's journey. Think about a time when there was criticism made of another medical specialty team related to patient care within your own circle. How did this feel to you?
- If the critique was explicitly expressed to the other team, who did this, and how was it done? If it was not expressed, do you think it should have been?
- What was the impact of the assessment on the ongoing collegial relationship between this team and yours?
- Did the critique influence ongoing patient care?
- Were there any constructive changes implemented after this event to optimise future care for that patient or others?
- A very destructive approach to discussing a harm event is to imply that 'YOU hurt MY patient'. This is a personal affront and implies that the patient is not shared by a clinical team. How can language like this be reframed to discuss decision-making while preserving relationships?
- When an ICU patient deteriorates under the care of one intensivist and then handoff occurs, this poses a challenge to address the situation without endangering the relationship with ICU colleagues. How can this inevitability be handled in a productive, sensitive way?

Standing Up to Bullying

... They (other specialties) are entitled to be where they are. *This* is where *we* are at that time, and I will work with you as much as I need to, to do it in the best interests of the patient. Whatever that takes. And if there is conflict, we just have to communicate about reasons for conflict. Not all wars need to be won on the first battle. That's probably a better way of phrasing it. And there are things that you can just live without, that are not going to cause any

problems. There are some things that you need to... I think, what I've learned is that, just, stand your ground a bit more, and not engage an adversarial opponent, but virtually stand up, and not be bullied around.

- There will always be different frames through which different medical specialties see the world. 'Choosing your battles' is an important concept for the intensivist, because often the war is being waged on several fronts! To continue with the analogy of 'battle', the intensivist needs to consider the big picture, the resources available, and the risk/benefit ratio of who is intervening and when. Most of all, they need to know where and how to take a stand to make these calls and be heard. Recall a situation where multiple teams were involved in the care of a complex patient. Who took priority, and how did the intensivist navigate and articulate this?
- How was it received by others, particularly those whose needs were not prioritised?
- What did you take away or learn from the interactions?
- When the first issue was addressed, how was the attention turned towards the next priority?
- In medicine and in life, the quote 'what you permit you promote' can resonate. How can you defuse tension and adversarial circumstances, advocate for yourself, and maintain professional relationships?
- Are there times when seeking advice or intervention from individuals outside of the ICU and outside of the conflict may be beneficial?

Conclusion

Intensivists of today need to be flexible and socially aware with other doctors. This is a deficiency of most trainees embarking on their ICU careers but is crucial to effectively manage complex patients. Being disingenuous or dismissive when evaluating patients outside of the ICU will quickly create animosity. Applying a 'my way or the highway' approach to ICU decisions will be poorly received amongst ICU colleagues. Tempering one's personal style for the unity of the ICU team is important. The ICU doctor needs to be malleable; the approach to consulting on a critical patient in the emergency room, inpatient ward, or location outside of the hospital needs to be nuanced and thoughtful. The skill sets, resources, and experience of these different doctors necessitate individualized approaches. These are not times for being sarcastic, laconic, or incomplete.

Being socially aware as an intensivist requires interpreting communication through multiple lenses. The surgeon will think differently than the infectious disease specialist, who will think differently than the intensivist. That makes managing a patient with septic shock from an abdominal abscess complicated. The task of managing the whole patient falls squarely on the shoulders of the intensivist. When differing plans or priorities are proposed, the intensivist must be the focused arbitrator. ICU patients are often clinically and emotionally shared by multiple clinical teams. Understanding the human element and mediating complexity are the crucial and rewarding charge of the intensivist.

Chapter 13
Different Performances, Kids are Special: Contemplating Pediatric ICU

Kelly Lyons

> *Children are the world's most valuable resource and its best hope for the future.*
>
> – *John F. Kennedy*

It is impossible to fully express the depth and meaning of a child's life to their loved ones. Many children rely on their families as surrogate decision-makers, and as such, the interplay of family dynamics and establishment of provider-family trust are essential to the delivery of pediatric critical care [1, 2]. As pediatric providers, we are responsible first and utmost to the child. At the same time, we must recognize the necessary balance when considering the potential role of the child in their own care as well as the role of their guardian in medical decision-making. Additionally, acknowledging the impact of the child's illness on the family's psychosocial construct is equally crucial. It is the formed partnerships with both the child and their support system that are at the core of pediatric critical care medicine. We are conductors of an orchestra in a performance (concert) that expands well outside of simply caring for a sick patient. This is what makes this specialty so different—kids are special.

When contemplating the physician-patient/family relationship, it is important to be mindful of the influence of society's viewpoint and potential misconceptions regarding pediatric critical illness during patient/family interactions. These perceptions may lead to potential guardian distress and may interfere with a family's understanding of the severity of their child's disease. A frequent misconception is that "children are generally healthy" and thereby not plagued by similar illnesses or risk of death due to lower overall mortality rates compared to adults. As pediatric

K. Lyons (✉)
University of Louisville Department of Pediatrics, Division of Critical Care,
and Norton Children's Medical Group, Louisville, KY, USA
e-mail: kelly.lyons.1@louisville.edu

137

critical care providers, part of our job is not only knowing the mortality rate is *NOT ZERO* but conveying severity of disease and providing compassionate end-of-life care for the dying child [3].

Historically, children are seen as the "hope" and the "future" amongst society. Children are songs yet to be sung, and as such it is likely to be unnatural for families to even fathom that their critically ill child may die. Further, many times we encounter cases where the future is "unknown"—we may have concerns for potential impairments for the child from their disease, but due to their age, they may "outgrow" or "improve" with rehabilitation or sometimes time. In those scenarios, it can be difficult to provide information and/or guide a family in shared decision-making, leading to potential stress for the provider. Discovering aspects of quality of life as determined by each family in those scenarios can help a provider unite with a family in the shared common goal of supporting their child.

As pediatric critical care providers, we each have found a calling to deliver the highest quality pediatric critical care to our respective patients. We are the conductors, and the critical care unit is our concert hall where the focus to create a healing environment is at the forefront. As emphasized, we should be mindful that while the child is our responsibility, we must respect their loved ones to provide the greatest care. The following quotations highlight the unique scenarios pediatric critical care providers face.

More Than Just the Patient

I think coming into it, you always think of the child, the patient. But I have grown to realise and appreciate the fact that it is more than just the patient. And I always say that now to the family. I say, 'I am your child's doctor but as much as I am here for him or her, I am also here for you'. Because I think that's a true statement.

- How does caring for a patient's family factor into your role as a pediatric ICU physician? Does it play a big part in your role, and if so, how?
- Thinking about your current ICU, describe ways you and your ICU team provide support to a patient's family during their child's ICU course?
- Do you feel it is important to explicitly tell a family "I am also here for you"?
- What are important aspects to building a trusting physician-family relationship, in addition to that formed with a child?
- Consider some of the barriers to having a good relationship with a child's family. What are some of the things you might do in preparation to both anticipate and overcome those things?
- Have you thought about how different family dynamics do/will affect the care you and your team provide?
- Consider your communication with families. What aspects of communication have worked well and strengthened that physician-family relationship vs. what aspects have not gone well and why?

- What are potential psychosocial stressors families can experience during a child's ICU stay? Do you consider these stressors in your approach to taking care of a child's family?

Communicating Severity of Illness to Families

We have a varying degree of acuity within our ICU and as far as the communication part of things go, parents, whether a kid just gets diagnosed with diabetes and they're going to be fine tomorrow or whether they're diagnosed with some devastating neurologic injury… There is no degree to that parent. It's all bad, right? So that's one of the things that I really like to make sure that people realise. If you don't know that this is the worst thing that's happened to their kid this day, and communicate that to them, then I think you've done everyone a disservice, and probably created some sort of anxiety or potential for there to be a lapse in understanding and trust.

- When you work in a place of high acuity, it may be difficult to regulate your response to less acute or less emergent patients and their families, and this quote speaks to that relativity. Do you think you can demonstrate empathy to families across the spectrum of patient acuity, and is this important for you?
- How do you and your team convey "acuity" of a child's illness to a family?
- You also have limited capacity in terms of your own personal energy and reserves to invest across all your patients and their families. How do you think you might identify and then navigate who "needs" you more than others?
- How do you currently empower families to seek support from you and your team? Do you think this is working? How could it be better?
- How do you and your team demonstrate compassion towards a child and their family?

Recognizing Family Perception of Illness

… You take care of every kid like they were your own. Some child comes in with a cold, you could be dismissive and roll your eyes, or you could, for that moment that you are interacting, show them that you understand that for them, this is the biggest thing that has ever happened. So, I try to do that…

- When handling high volume of patients, how do you treat and recognize each scenario as the "biggest thing that has ever happened" for that child and family?
- Handling high acuity patients, while rewarding, can also be taxing for an ICU team. How do you process and support your own emotional wellness while treating "the worst" scenarios for patients and families?

- How do you try to not "be dismissive" of a family's concerns for their child?
- Do you agree or disagree that pediatric intensivists should "take care of every kid like they were your own"? Why do you agree or disagree?
- How do you and your team work together with families who may have differences and not share your same view or perception of their child's illness?

Balancing Hope for Families

I had a parent whose child was going to die and they were making a decision about withdrawing life-sustaining therapies. And on some level they understood that the patient was not going to make it through this and on another level, they were waiting for a miracle to happen...

- Consider the word "miracle"—what connotation does that word have for you? Have you encountered families who are hopeful for "a miracle"? If so, what particularly stands out in those family encounters as compared to others?
- How can we help families cope with the balance between hope and the sometimes unfortunate realities of end-of-life scenarios such as described in the quote?
- How do you cope with your own processing of hope when in the face of severe conditions encountered in the PICU?
- In pediatrics, families may mention or potentially feel the notion of "giving up"—how do you and your ICU team help support a family reframe in those moments?

Managing Family Dynamics at End of Life

I'd say one of the hardest parts of being a PICU doctor is bridging the medicine with the family dynamic. I had a dying child's mother say to me recently 'All I know is that I'm supposed to never give up on him. I'm his mother and I was put on this planet to be his strength'. How do you turn that beautiful reality into a conversation about dying well?

- Considering the comment made by the mother, how would you respond?
- What are ways that you and your ICU team could provide support to this mother?
- When considering end-of-life scenarios, what potential support services would you consider involving at your respective institutions?
- Consider the final two words—"dying well"—what does that mean to you? Is the concept of "dying well" important in your approach and discussions with a family at end of life?
- Think back to a scenario where you have provided guidance for a family with a child at end of life. How did you approach and guide that family? How did the family dynamics play a role in the guidance you provided?

Communicating with Families Under Extenuated Circumstances

And the hard thing is that some of our parents don't have adult coping mechanisms. Some of them are not adults; you know we have… I can think of one patient in particular…. The kid had congenital heart disease; very severe; and the mother was 14. And I was like, 'I have a 13-year-old (at home). How would I explain this'? Because you are always taught to explain things to the parent, not the grandparent; but this girl is like my son's age, and she is having to care for a baby who has, like, very severe… And her mother, the grandparent is my age, and so I am looking at her; realising that that's not the right thing; it's not her baby…

- Having a parent who is a child themselves is not an uncommon scenario in the pediatric ICU, but is it something you have thought about?
- What specific skills or tools do you think you need to cultivate within your repertoire to be able to communicate with a child who has assumed an adult role in the context of being a parent?
- What are the barriers and enablers to effective communication in this circumstance?
- What do you think you need to consider when conveying adult themes like morbidity and mortality to a child-parent?
- How do you balance the role of extended family members, such as the grandparent mentioned, in this circumstance?
- When considering discussions such as above, is it vital to consider what is important/how a caregiver likes to make medical decisions? If so, why?
- What are potential psychosocial stressors that the mother in this scenario may be experiencing, and how can you and your team help to alleviate those stressors?

Giving Families Grace

There is nothing 'natural' about being a parent and having to make decisions about a serious illness or possible death of your child. Those are conversations that we are meant to have about our elderly family members at the expected end of their lives. I think it's important to start by giving families grace. To tell them that it's OKAY to not know how to feel or what to say. Our job is to join them on this journey.

- How do you and your team help "join" a family on their "journey" regarding their child's illness?
- Consider the last time you gave a family "grace"—what stood out and was particular about that case? How can you apply the same compassion towards your future families?

- When considering shared decision-making, how do you help a family deal with the "unnaturalness" of making difficult decisions surrounding their child's illness, particularly decisions involving end of life?
- This quote highlights potential societal views surrounding different age populations, particularly pertaining to end of life. How do you (if at all) take into consideration society's viewpoint on pediatric critical illness and particularly end-of-life care of pediatrics when caring for a dying child?
- Have you ever told a family "It's OKAY to not know how to feel or what to say"? If so, when and what were the circumstances? Did you find the phrasing helped support that family?

Shared Decision-Making with Families

In my patients, it's a rarity that I can talk to my patient and ask them what they want me to do, or offer them. Most often I am going to a parent, I partner with a parent, to help them understand what the right thing is for their loved one, their child. So I think that those dynamics make things a little bit different. There is an expectation. There's something special about children. There's this "potential" for children. I look at my patient who is nine months old, and wonder, 'Could this kid be the president some day?

- Consider the surrogacy of decision-making in the care of children. Have you thought about the implications for your practice in the pediatric ICU?
- This quotation refers to the "right thing to do". How do you interpret what that means, and do you think that it would always necessarily be the same for both you and the parents?
- Can you think of situations where it might be difficult for you to define the "right thing to do"? What do you think your approach would be in those circumstances?
- Are you familiar with the legalities around the age of consent in the country where you practice?
- This quotation discusses how not all children can participate in their own decision-making, but for those who can, do you feel the child has a role in their own decision-making?
- This quotation emphasizes the "potential" and "expectations" for children, how do you interpret what that means, and does that also influence your approach to decision-making for children?
- Prognostication in children can be difficult. Consider your approach to how you discuss prognostication with a child and family. What is important to include in those discussions, where are those discussions occurring, and who is a part of those discussions?
- When considering shared decision-making, how does the child's quality of life play a role for that family, and/or should quality influence medical decisions being made?

- This quotation emphasizes the concept of "partnering" with a parent—what does that look like? Is "partnering" important in shared medical decision-making, and if so, why?

The Parent Intensivist

I'd say that one of the most special and emotional challenges of working in a pediatric ICU as opposed to and adult ICU is acceptance. Acceptance that PICU doctors are often parents of healthy children and can see their own child reflected in their patients. Acceptance that many people see our calling as unnatural and heartbreaking. Being a parent of healthy children, I turn these emotions into gratitude and importance. I don't take my child's health for granted. I don't dismiss or minimize the anguish of my patients' families. That's the beauty of this profession and not everyone gets it.

- Consider the quote's reference to "acceptance"—do you resonate with that notion of "acceptance" as expressed within the quote? Why or why not?
- Reflect on how your own experience of either being a parent or not influences your practice within the ICU. Does it play a role when interacting with patients and families? If so, how?
- As the quote alludes to "many people see our calling as unnatural"—take a moment to consider why that is. Have you experienced or had others express similar concerns to you when talking about your profession as a pediatric intensivist?
- What are your "special" challenges that you find separates the care in the PICU from the adult ICU?
- How do you like to describe your profession to those close to you? Do you try to minimize your experiences? Do you find it difficult to explain the details of your profession as a pediatric intensivist to others? If so, why?
- When taking care of a patient, how do you manage potential reflections/associations that patient may have to a loved one of yours? Does it impact your care?

Impact of Pediatric Intensive Care on Childhood Mortality

One of the stressors that I perceive is that while that mortality rate should be 3%, that that mortality rate doesn't maintain itself. It is 3% because we work really hard, and we think really hard, and I think sometimes pediatric providers can be lulled into a complacency about that. They don't realise that our efforts actually matter. Like if we stood back and just let kids do what they do, the mortality rate isn't going to go from 3 to 40%, the mortality rate is gonna go from like 3 to 8% or something like that… If we do things right, we absolutely can help kids get better; but they don't just get better on their own.

- This quote speaks to the burden on pediatric ICU doctors around the fact that they don't expect children to die, and so there is an added pressure to ensure they survive the critical illness that resulted in their ICU admission. And sometimes they do, and sometimes they don't. As a doctor working with children, reflect on experiencing the death of a patient.
- Do you think it's different for doctors working with adults where death is perhaps a more permissible and acceptable outcome?
- Can you consider that the death of an elderly matriarch might be just as traumatic for those involved in patient care? Why do you think that is?
- This quotation comments "they don't realize that our efforts actually matter" referring to pediatric providers. How do you interpret this, and why would pediatric providers be more "complacent" about pediatric mortality?
- How do you explain to a family the severity of their child's illness and prognostication? Does the pediatric mortality rate mentioned in the quotation influence your discussion on severity of illness?
- Does the pediatric mortality rate change the impact of a child's death for you and/or your ICU team?
- Do you believe in the notion that children get better quicker and therefore that notion influences expectations for recovery?
- Do you feel the stress of "working really hard" to maintain the low pediatric mortality rate? Does this impact your patient-family interactions? Does this impact your job satisfaction?

Different than Adult: Processing the Death of a Child

Death in the PICU is way different than the MICU. I've been a doctor for both. It starts with knowing that the longer an adult is in the ICU, then more likely they are to die and the opposite is true for children. So when the death of a child approaches, all sorts of emotions surface. As a PICU doctor you can be confronted with belligerent refusal to 'give up'. You expect a family to struggle with denial.

Some of the most beautiful moments I've had the honour of being present for are when a wise grandparent, who has experienced death and can lean on their life experiences, takes the lead.

- Have you ever experienced being confronted with the "refusal to give up" notion as represented by the quotation above? If so, when?
- Consider families you have cared for where those "beautiful moments" during end of life care occurred for their children. What stands out to you from those moments? What particularly about those families do you remember? Is it if a particular family member, ritual, ceremony, memory making, etc.?
- As the quote highlights, many emotions arise during end-of-life care of a child. Consider some of the emotions you have seen families express, and consider the

ways you and your team supported the family. What emotions were you, as the provider, potentially experiencing?
- How do you cope with the death of a pediatric patient? How does your ICU team support each other following the death of a pediatric patient?

Recognizing the Importance of Grief and Bereavement Support for Families

It wasn't the child's death that was so profoundly impactful, it was the mother's grief that was more impactful. It was her sobbing, you know 'How do I go on; what do I do; and where do I go'?…that type of loss; recognizing that the families are going home to laundry baskets, and to toys and to dreams that have just all of a sudden, been ended.

- Consider the resources within your ICU and home institution—what grief and bereavement support are provided for families and by who?
- Do you feel there is a role of the pediatric intensive care team to provide ongoing bereavement support to families? If yes, why? If no, why?
- Have you or a member of your intensive care team attended a funeral for a patient? What stood out to you about that experience? Did it change your practice within the ICU?
- Have your own personal experiences of loss of a loved one influence your approach to grieving families?
- What aspects of postmortem care offered by your institution? Is memory making incorporated and if so, what items?
- Postmortem, what resources can we provide for spiritual support to families?
- How can we incorporate specific cultural beliefs of a family into postmortem care for the patient?

Conclusion

To thrive as a pediatric intensivist is to become absorbed in a complex symphony. The field presents many unique challenges from addressing family perception of their child's illness to managing expectations regarding outcomes to providing compassionate end-of-life care. An overarching theme of the importance of the child/family/provider relationship, particularly in areas such as shared decision-making, conveying severity of illness, and aspects of end-of-life care, was emphasized. Equally as stressed was the recognition that "…this is the biggest thing that has ever happened…" for families with children in the intensive care unit. While our perceptions may not always align with parental views of acuity, being mindful to approach each patient encounter with the same dedication and fervor is vital. Lastly, the knowledge to convey that "kids can get sick too" and employ that notion during discussions with families regarding the "future" and potential uncertainties is valuable.

As we contemplate these resounding themes, think back, and consider your individual and your team's approach to each of the proposed questions. By continuing to foster a growth mindset in learning from our past experiences while creating safe environments for our own future wellness, we can promote resiliency within our field. Remembering that as important as it is that we set the "stage", we accept that we are playing along to the child's song. The unique scenarios posed by the pediatric population and their loved ones, while yes sometimes challenging, are ultimately an honour to take care of and one that pediatric critical care providers do not take for granted.

References

1. Dennis D, van Heerden P, Khanna R, Knott C, Zhang S, Calhoun A. The different challenges in being an adult versus a pediatric intensivist. Crit Care Explor. 2022;4(3):e0654. https://doi.org/10.1097/CCE.0000000000000654. PMID: 35261983; PMCID: PMC8893297
2. Wheeler DS, Dewan M, Maxwell A, Riley CL, Stalets EL. Staffing and workforce issues in the pediatric intensive care unit. Transl Pediatr. 2018;7(4):275–83. https://doi.org/10.21037/tp.2018.09.05. PMID: 30460179; PMCID: PMC6212383
3. Dryden-Palmer K, Garros D, Meyer EC, Farrell C, Parshuram CS. Care for dying children and their families in the PICU: promoting clinician education, support, and resilience. Pediatr Crit Care Med. 2018;19(8S):S79–85. https://doi.org/10.1097/PCC.0000000000001594.

Chapter 14
Leading the Choir: Contemplating Communicating with Your Own Team

Zena Leah Harris ⓘD

> *If your actions inspire others to dream more, learn more, do more and become more, you are a leader.*
>
> *– John Quincy Adams*

Team communication is critical for success in any and every way, and how the members of a team respond to each other inside and outside a crisis will define outcomes. Using a song as the metaphor for a healthcare crisis, the intensivist's role of 'leading the choir to sing' means being able to help each team member to identify their own strengths and limitations enabling them to proactively navigate challenges together, hitting the right notes at the right time whilst maintaining the tune—or the health—of the team itself. We no longer live in an era of a singular hierarchy or a singular team. We are interconnected and interprofessional and span gender, race, age and experiences. Our differences make us stronger but only if we can harness that thought diversity. In many ways a successful leader is one that can quickly assess the culture of the team and identify activities and approaches that will unite them. Assigning tasks, asking people to bring questions to the group for everyone to consider and address and asking people what their goals are for the shift, the week or the month together are all techniques to help bring all your team members together. Making feedback and celebrating intellectual diversity a goal for the rotation help make this conversation more comfortable to others. With time, it will become intuitive, but trainees need to see this behaviour role modelled and embraced by their leaders. Don't contemplate communication—insist on effective communication, build mechanisms to ensure everyone feels safe to speak up, and include everyone in the conversation over the course of rounds.

Z. L. Harris (✉)
Dell Medical School at The University of Texas at Austin, Austin, TX, USA

Dell Children's Medical Center, Austin, TX, USA
e-mail: zena.harris@austin.utexas.edu

D. Dennis et al. (eds.), *Contemplating the Role of an Intensive Care Doctor*, https://doi.org/10.1007/978-3-031-92766-9_14

147

Shared Prospective Understanding of Poor Prognosis

Respondent	**I realised recently that the Residents don't have that knowledge yet.**
Interviewer	**They think they are going to save everyone?**
Respondent	**Yes. Not everyone, but much more so. So let's say I'm 95% correct [predicting a negative outcome]; they may be 50% correct. So, to them, I've realised—and this is part of their burnout—they really think that we can save them… To me, it was so obvious that I didn't think I [needed to] tell them. And I realised … they don't know. So, I think I could do a better job of being very explicit in that, so that they at least hear it, and can do what they can do with that information… so, it's not as surprising.**

- Some doctors come into medicine with unreasonable expectations around their capacity to impact the certainty of survival of their patients. Whilst you will always want to maximise a patient's potential, have you ever been disappointed by an unanticipated poor patient outcome?
- Have you ever sensed that a more senior colleague expected a poor patient outcome and was less surprised than you when it transpired?
- If a colleague was to prognosticate a patient outcome differently to you, how do you think you would respond?
- Have you ever sensed that a more senior colleague did not expect a poor patient outcome and was just as surprised as you when it transpired?
- If so, what did you notice about the way they coped with the situation? If not, why do you think that they had this understanding before you did?
- Have you ever thought about how important hope is? We find ourselves in medicine so data-driven and fact-based and are taught to realise that hope is not a strategy. And yet, it is hard not to hope that the predictions will fail, and the patient will be the one to 'beat the odds'.
- When someone tells you the ending of a book when you have just started reading the book, how does it make you feel? Would you feel the same way if the outcome of a patient was shared with you the same way? How would it change your approach to your colleagues? The bedside nurse? The family? The way you support each other?
- How important is it for all of us to be working with the same medical model for a patient? Do surgeons have the same model as the intensivists? Aren't these different approaches important in bringing out the best care from all teams?

Shared Decision-Making to Stop

Another thing that I have learnt from my practice that I have tried to impart on others, is for example, in a resuscitation, to ask everybody in the room if they are comfortable stopping and that they can sleep at night as well as I can. So that if someone says, "I don't know why we did that resuscitation", I will say that "I also need to sleep at night", and it is important that we take our emotional well-being into account and as a leader, we need to take into account everybody's well-being.

- As a team leader, it can sometimes feel very lonely at the top of the hierarchical tree of decision-making. Shared decision-making does not negate the power or respect you garner from your team as team leader and may actually enhance it. Have you ever asked your team to contribute to a shared decision related to emergent care?
- If so, how did it impact your feelings about the episode? If not, imagine how it might impact your emotions.
- This quote also speaks to our new understanding of situational awareness, as something that you either have or do not have, rather than something to 'lose' or 'gain' in the middle of an acute event. Sometimes you will have a keen awareness that you do not have all the information related to the people in the room at any one time, and there may be people present who could offer other opinions and input when you are at the limit of your own. Think of an acute event where someone suggested something that worked well. How do you think the leader was able to elicit that contribution?
- How do you enable people to speak up during an emergent event and be comfortable in doing so?
- Have you ever witnessed an action and not felt you could speak up?
- Think of when this might be challenging, and what you might do to facilitate it in those circumstances?
- The quote above assumes that stopping resuscitation was the right thing to do. How might this be different if there was clearly a reversible process and in fact resuscitation should be continued?
- The leader of a resuscitation is usually the most senior person present and may not be the person who knows the patient and their issues best. How might a team leader designate someone as a 'co-pilot' to help them?
- It is very natural for us to blame ourselves for a faulty decision when something goes wrong or when a desired outcome cannot be obtained. Often, younger members of the team—nurses and therapists—will feel their actions led to the code event. How might debriefing the event help after stopping the resuscitation?
- We share decision-making when the patient is being treated. Doesn't it seem the next extension to share decision-making to end treatment?

Second Guessing Prognosis Retrospectively

I have a couple of trainees who were beating themselves up about something that they missed, but the child was already dead when he got here. And there were beating themselves up over things that they had missed and I had to be like, "you know, there is a lesson; there is an important lesson in here for you; but the lesson is not about these details here because that was already all done; nothing you did impacted the outcome for this child; we need to be clear on this; you didn't do anything to harm this child; but there are things that you can learn here, that might save another child. It might help you save a child really meaningfully, in a different way. So don't focus on this outcome because this outcome was not your fault; it's not your burden; it's not".

- When doctors self-reflect on patient care, they often rightly focus on their own role in the patient journey. One of the important things that experienced intensivists have shared is that both poor and positive outcomes precipitate significant teachable moments for those involved. Consider a patient who deteriorated under your care. What did you learn? What did you change for next time?
- How did you draw these conclusions? For example, did you seek out someone to walk through the scenario with, and was that a fruitful experience; or did you do it on your own? Based on how it went, how would you work through an event next time to maximise your personal growth?
- How did you pass this knowledge forward to your peers and co-workers?
- Our medical vision is always 20/20 the following day. Many of the decisions we must make are done in a vacuum without all the data and history. It is only with time and investigation are details often made available. How can you then be held responsible for doing your best with limited information?
- We often presume that the patient that has presented to us was in their usual state of 'good health' when, in actuality, the patient had something physiologically very wrong that was not yet recognised. The patient, in fact, was a ticking time bomb. What about their presentation supports that idea?
- While patterns of disease are very important to recognise, how can we avoid practicing by pattern recognition and develop the ability to be more proactive in our patient's care?
- What does it mean to be 'at fault'? Isn't there an implication that you had the ability to intervene and change the outcome and you didn't and hence you are at fault? If you are managing a problem that has presented to you, how can you be 'at fault'?

Transparency

I want to be transparent about them [errors] because I've made my mistakes, and people should know about them so they don't have to make the same mistake—they might do a variation and a new mistake, but then they can tell someone about it. I think the people who are involved need to be involved. If there is a nursing error because something was… a device was handled in such a way that it is not in concert with our established practices… And that resulted in a bad event, they should be responsible for that. If there is a surgical misadventure, the surgeon should be responsible for that. Pediatric Intensivists should not be held responsible for a surgical mishap. Vice versa applies as well. And that's important. We need to understand where the error was and what the event was, so that we can have a collective unified mental model of what the problem is and how to reverse it. If you know what the problem is, then you can devise a solution that's specific to that problem, which is high yield.

- This quote not only reflects a clear sense of what is required for transparency, but it also highlights a fundamental tenant that repeating the same mistake should not be tolerated. In other words, it's not the mistake that is the problem, but it's the possibility that the cause of the mistake is not remediated in a way that is prophylactic for next time. Have you heard the aphorism 'Mistakes are puzzles to be solved rather than crimes to be punished'? It may be easy to apply this adage to others, but how frequently do you apply it to yourself?
- The opposite of success is not failure. We fail at something every day. The opposite of success is mediocrity and not caring. You cared, you tried, and you failed. Being able to share that mistake—that failure—is critical in your own reflection and growth as well as others. How do you teach others not to repeat a mistake you have made?
- Critical to transparency is being sure we are speaking the same medical language. A surgeon not putting something in their operative report may reflect that they don't see the events that transpired in the operative suite as anything more than a variation on approach, while the medical team or anaesthesia team may see it differently. Can you think of a way you might query a colleague about events or details without having it come across as criticising or antagonising?
- When I see someone doing something or ordering something that would not have been a part of my approach to a problem, I often ask, 'Can you share more with me why this is something you are ordering? It never would have occurred to me to have managed this situation this way'? Can you think of a time this might have been a valuable approach to a scenario? Might this have made the report seem more transparent?

Being Questioned

If you can see something that looks like it's a high probability or eventuality, it would be finding your way to constructively say, "Are you sure you want to do that? Have you thought about… why don't we have a chat to someone else and see what they think"? … I think "Are you sure"? is the most loaded and important question in intensive care. As soon as someone asks, "Are you sure"? You shouldn't be.

- There are two players within this scenario—the person delivering the challenge and the person receiving it. Consider both. How do you enable one of your team members to challenge an action in the moment by speaking up to the person involved?
- What steps have you already enacted to facilitate your team to speak up to you?
- Think of the last time it happened. Can you reflect on the impact of that communication in terms of what worked well, and what would you change the next time you had that experience?
- If no one has ever spoken up to you, has there ever been a time when you wished they had?
- Think of a time when you 'spoke up' to a colleague to question a decision or action in the moment. How did you do that, and how was it received?
- With hindsight, what worked well, and what would you change the next time you had that experience?
- The corollary of 'Are you sure'? is 'Because I said so'! It is as equally important to be able to navigate dogma as it is personal patterns of practice. Have you ever had this happen to you?

Asking for Help

Speaking up, but also having the confidence to say, "I'm not comfortable at this point in time". So, recognising one's limitations and being comfortable to admit that you have limitations. You know, we've all got limitations. I run patients past my senior consultants when I need to… "What do you think about this? This is what I'm thinking…", so I think that's important.

- In the high acuity environment of intensive care, it is highly likely that you will be involved in situations from time to time where co-workers might presume you to have more knowledge or skill than you feel you own. Some of that will be due to a lack of confidence because you perceive yourself to have insufficient practical experience or exposure; some will be because you are genuinely completely out of your depth. The maxim of 'Faking it until you make it' may have placed you in this position, while the 'Imposter syndrome' may make it difficult for you to navigate the moment. How do you think you will be able to recognise and articulate your own limitations in an emergent situation?

- What traits do the people you admire most in our field have? They certainly must ask for help and while experts in one domain, not be experts in all. How do they reach out for help?
- As an intensivist you are expected to know 1,000 things about 100,000 diseases! There is no way to know it all. How do you stay current in your learning?
- Have you ever been called in the middle of the night and asked by a colleague for help or advice? How did it make you feel? Did it change how you feel about reaching out for help?
- When you start a night shift, do you look at the team you are on with and assess what skills and strengths they bring to the team? Do you look to see who your most senior people are in-house (surgery, anaesthesia) in case you need back-up?
- Have you ever called a colleague and just let them know that you have a sick patient and that you might need them?

Followership

… A good leader can make a good follower as well… That's being able to take direction but also feedback information appropriately. And most of the time we will be the leaders, but sometimes… it might be that I will say (to a trainee), "you're going to run this, you take the leadership" and then hopefully I can display some followership and do my bit…

- The value of good followership within a team can never be underestimated. As a team leader, what traits do you look for in a good follower?
- How do you encourage and enhance these qualities?
- Have you ever taken on a followership role to explicitly model your own expectations around good followership?
- If so, what did this feel like; what did it teach you; and what was the impact on the leader and the team? If not, is it something you could do; or do you perceive there to be barriers that would need to be overcome?
- One of my favourite images involves Canadian geese: their V-formation reveals the strength of sharing the lead, and when the lead goose gets tired, it moves to the back and drafts from the bird in front. Can you use this as an example of how you work in the ICU? When do you lead and when do you draft?
- A famous Lewis Carroll quote is 'if you don't know where you are going, any road will get you there'. What does that mean to you in terms of following and leading?

Team Member Seeking Feedback on Performance

We are all sensitive to one another. Because you are not going to be like, "Oh I would have… I totally disagree…" You know, your goal is not to make the other person feel worse… If someone comes to me, and when I listen, I hear something, and (I'll say), "I might have done this, but I don't think it would have changed your outcome". Right, like I might have intubated an hour later, or an hour sooner, or I might have used this drug not that drug; but then finishing it with, "I don't know if it would have changed the outcome". So, like talking through the case…

- This quote reflects empathy and kindness towards someone seeking feedback on their performance. Think about the last time you offered support to a co-worker. Can you relate to this approach? What was your experience like?
- Consider what you think you need to provide to a co-worker. It may be clinical expertise, emotional support or just time and space for them to reflect. How do you explore what the help-seeker really needs? Your style may be different depending on your relationship with them.
- Giving feedback is an art, and finding the right time to give someone feedback is equally important. Do you have the habit of sharing feedback with the members of your team—junior and senior?
- When you give feedback, do you ever then ask the person you shared feedback with to also give you feedback on your performance?
- Can you remember a time when feedback was given to you that was revealing and important to you? Can you remember what made that conversation so impactful?
- Normalising feedback is important. Have you ever asked someone to watch you do a procedure and give your real-time feedback?

Cultivating a Workplace Culture That Normalises Checking in

I think the culture of a busy ICU is such that we are meant to, I guess, just cope and deal with things. I think that's how you get through your training, and that's probably subliminally the message to juniors as well. I think we probably don't check enough on, especially junior, staff. For us it becomes more and more routine to see bad stuff day by day, and I just accept that as part of intensive care. And I think the culture of ICU is probably not one where… it is not kind of touchy-feely, although it probably should be a bit more that way—where help should be readily on offer—I guess there should be a system where we can check in with each other and with junior staff and with nursing staff more readily.

I was coming onto service on Thursday, but on Monday I knew that one of my partners… We had lost a patient that we all loved and were very invested in; and it was hard… And I texted him, and I said, "Hey I just wanted to check in on how you are doing; I know it's been a hard week". And I think our whole group is like that. I think it's a culture that we have cultivated within our division specifically, where we all check-in on each other.

- Consider the workplace culture within your intensive care. Do you believe that co-workers check in with each other both within their profession and across other professional groups?
- Do you currently make a point of explicitly checking in on your peers? Your mentors? Your juniors? Other team members who are not doctors?
- How successful have you been so far in your career in considering and then navigating your concern for those who work with you?
- Is there anything you specifically do to express your appreciation for other staff within your workplace?
- Has a colleague ever overtly done something for you that positively impacted your well-being at work? What was that, and how did it make you feel?
- What did you learn from that, and did you pass it forward to someone else?

  How do you positively impact the culture of your workplace in terms of staff well-being?

Checking in with Peers

Most of it is pre-emptive. If this had happened to me, I would feel broken; I would feel injured; I would feel distraught; I would feel stressed; I would feel scared. And if you can pre-emptively identify how (an event) would impact you, you can generally address it head-on (with others).

- Checking in with near peers can be a rewarding experience, as you may have a comparatively closer connection in terms of relatability. Perhaps you have encountered a similar issue recently on your own journey; perhaps you are just better able to place yourself in their shoes because you have the same level of clinical exposure. Do you think you are able to empathise with your peers, and they with you?
- What are the barriers to feeling empathy for a peer, and how might you overcome them?
- What are the barriers to identifying a peer who is in distress, and how might you address them proactively?
- Does supporting a peer impact negatively on your own confidence?
- Can you imagine training in an environment where you were the solo fellow?

- If you had to build a community to train in, practice with and work in, what would it look like? Who would your peers be? What interprofessional peers do you rely on the most?
- Think about your tiers of peers? What makes someone a close peer?

Checking in Upwardly

[From a junior consultant]: 'People who are junior to me, or more junior faculty, I am much more open to checking in with them and seeing how they are doing. The people who are my level, or higher, I feel very uncomfortable checking in to see if they're doing okay'.

[From a senior consultant]: 'The number of times something has happened, it's been rare for somebody to ask me how I was doing. Very, very rare'.

- It is often difficult to support co-workers or mentors who are perceived to be above you in the hierarchy of control. This may be because you hold a perception of the omniscience of those people or a presumption that they are unperturbed by the work they do, as they've been navigating the role for a long time before you came along! It may also feel disrespectful for you to presume that they too might need to be supported. Consider these people. Do you ever offer support to them as part of your engagement in the relationship?
- What are the barriers to identifying a senior colleague who is in distress, and how might you address them proactively?
- If you were concerned for a senior colleague, how would you broach the subject of support?
- What are the barriers to feeling empathy for a senior colleague, and how might you overcome them?
- The hierarchy of medicine implies that the most senior person is the most knowledgeable and also the one with the most professional life experience. They are 'survivors' and have developed coping mechanisms to deal with adversity. Have you ever asked a more senior colleague how they cope? How they navigate the challenges we face in this career?
- Vulnerability is an emotion that often makes us more authentic. Can you remember a more senior colleague revealing their vulnerabilities? Crying with a family? Sharing with the team that a decision is difficult?

If a senior colleague asked for help, would you know what to do? Who would you turn to?

Providing Bespoke Support—Individual Differences

(The) ability to recognise what checking on their mental health or emotional management of the situation is. So for some people, that would be, just having a chat to, "Are you okay"? Other people that would maybe have a more coffee with; other people who…. Someone else you might be a bit more concerned about, you might have a formal debriefing process for that… so I think (intensivists) have got a significant role (and) a very difficult role, in many cases.

They were like, "I wish people would just stop talking; just stop asking me if I'm okay; I will talk to you if I'm not okay". They were just a very private person. So, I've tried to be very mindful of that as I have moved forward. Some people like to talk and process verbally; some people don't; but I think, at least showing that you care. Because I think if you went on and pretended like nothing had happened, and go on about life, then you're not doing your job as a mentor.

- Consider the personal relationships you have with your work colleagues. Some of these people you will know well; others you will know at a surface level. If you were concerned for one of them, consider how this might look quite different depending on who they were and what you know of them. Choose a few of them, and consider how you would broach the subject of support in each case.
- Think about the time and place of the initial suggestion; think about how you might follow that up.
- When checking in with your co-workers, how would you or do you manage the perception of stigma around them seeking professional support?
- Do you understand the services that are accessible for help-seekers needing to access formal support within your own institutions?
- Do you understand the services that are accessible for help-seekers needing to access formal support within your own state or country?
- Have there been times where your gender, or age, or race may have hindered your ability to support a colleague?
- Have there been times when you have used an 'intermediary' to help offer support to a colleague?
- Have you ever pre-discussed how the members of your team want to be supported? Asked people on the first day of a rotation together not only what their goals for your time together are but how you can best support them in decision-making and in poor outcome scenarios? If not, might you think about doing that moving forward?

Conclusion

The quotes shared in this chapter, along with their contemplation dot points, are designed to enable essential conversations. All of us, at some point, wished we had a guide or map to help navigate the difficult conversations that present to us. This is the hope of this chapter—to be a guide to better communication. There are a few important points about communication to keep in mind as you grow in your commitment to taking care of your team. Communication is as much what is said and what is intuited. There is a famous quote from Simon Sinek, 'Hearing is listening to what is said. Listening is hearing what isn't said'. It is not enough to be in a room and share ideas or be a sounding board. To truly communicate and have meaningful conversation, you must truly listen. It is also important to consider the lens through which the other person is coming from. This is not always easy to do but essential as we build our teams with diverse members, from different backgrounds and with different roles. Seeing a conversation or event through the other person's point of view allows you to appreciate the differences between you. Crossing that divide is how you garner trust and respect and prepare your team to take on the next challenge together.

Part IV
Mastering Aerial Acrobatics

Foreword: How to Be a Trapeze Artist

Bertrand Guidet

> Life is either always a tight-rope or a featherbed. Give me a tight-rope. (Edith Wharton)

What are the similarities between a trapeze artist and an intensive care (ICU) physician? They both work hard in dangerous conditions and train constantly. They need trust in their partners and work as part of a team. When a trapeze artist fails in his performance, he falls. When an ICU physician fails, the patient might die, with enormous personal consequences for the doctor (for example, litigation, culpability, burn-out and so on) and of course the patient. The high cognitive burden may hinder the personal life and future career of the trapeze artist and the doctor. Like the trapeze artist, intensive care doctors need to maintain the right distance from the patient and their relatives, but also within the ICU team. If the distance is poorly judged (too short or too large), the trapeze artist could fall and the doctor might quit.

How should we be promoting intensive care medicine to be attractive to young doctors? How do we take care of health care workers with the hypothesis that a happy junior physician will provide good quality medicine? These are some of the pertinent questions addressed in this part of the book. We discuss how to climb the ropes and flourish as a performer when there may be personal doubt; how to be accepting of unanticipated career challenges; and how to install safety nets for yourself to catch you if you falter.

Yes, ICU is stressful and may generate fatigue and daily questioning of work-life balance. Yes, our specialty is very demanding: dealing with life and death, requiring a wide medical knowledge, expertise at performing procedures, an ability to communicate with the team, the patient and their surrogates, a constant need to update knowledge and long hours, including after-hours work. However, all these potential drawbacks are in fact the beauty and the wonder of our specialty. Intensive care is inclusive and holistic. It mobilizes diagnostic ability, procedural skills, teamwork and ethics. We take care of patients from different backgrounds and socio-economic status. We work with a group of people with different education levels. Our specialty enables us to open our mind and to have a broader view of society and challenges. We have unique opportunities to tackle fundamental questions.

The ICU-stay is only a small part of the trajectory of the patient in hospital. The journey starts before ICU admission to after hospital discharge. To optimize the patient pathway, we need collaboration—sometimes even negotiation—with other specialties: surgeons for high-risk surgical patients, haematologists for patients with myeloma, emergency physicians for elderly multimorbid patients and so on. We act as a bridge between specialties to optimize post-ICU care. For elderly patients in particular, the involvement of geriatricians should be promoted.

We treat very unstable patients with a high risk of making errors. The root causes of adverse events are often systemic, and individual blame should be de-emphasized. A non-punishing policy should be promoted within the ICU and by the institution. Formal discussion in morbidity mortality reviews is very helpful. Mitigation measures that helped prevent serious consequences should be acknowledged and learnt from. Feeling anxious—having a kind "stage fright", like actors before a performance—is common before starting a high-stakes procedure, like a difficult intubation. These feelings should be accepted or even promoted because they demonstrate the concern we hold for our duty and for the responsibility to and for the patients we are caring for.

Much of what we should consider when communicating with patients and their families has already been explored in Part III. Death is part of our daily practice: how best to inform the family, and how information is shared among the team members? A bit of dissension is welcome since it means that it allows people to express different points of view. A dignified death prevents complicated grief and potential conflict. The climate and culture of the ICU team are key. The main values and ethos of the unit need to be shared and acknowledged by all the team. Fear of being stigmatized leads to isolation and stress. We are trusted by patients and their relatives. In response, we need to be competent, available and transparent. As humans, we all seek personal rewards, but need to learn to say, "we collectively performed well". We need to congratulate each other. We need to express gratitude to others, and they will provide the same in return. We need to build a culture of mutual respect and solidarity within the team.

A friendly and professional atmosphere will allow us to express our doubts and difficulties. The best reward is when patients and their family say, "Thank you".

Chapter 15
Learning to Climb the Ropes – Shadows of Doubt: Contemplating Self-Care

Eileen Tay

> *Keep your face to the sunshine and you cannot see a shadow.*
>
> *– Helen Keller*

This chapter relates to self-care and provides some incredible, profound insights into the myriads of reactions doctors working in the ICUs find themselves experiencing, both professionally and personally. It was a challenge to transform these kernels of truth into something that may be helpful for readers and organizational leaders to reflect upon to increase their overall capacity to cope and manage difficult thoughts and feelings at both an individual level during their career and a systems level. I hope the comments, information and reflective exercises that have been incorporated into this chapter do some justice to the candid and courageous contributions from the original research participants.

Every one of us learned to climb the ropes at some stage, all with shadows of doubt. I find myself as a mid-stage career psychiatrist wearing more and more hats, and the ones I increasingly enjoy are those of an educator, supervisor and mentor, and I also hope that those at mid- or late-stage careers will embrace these roles for the next generation of doctors.

E. Tay (✉)
Medical School, University of Western Australia, Perth, Western Australia

RANZCP Faculty of Forensic Psychiatry and Faculty of Psychotherapy, Melbourne, VIC, Australia
e-mail: eileen.tay@health.wa.gov.au

© The Author(s), under exclusive license to Springer Nature Switzerland AG 2025
D. Dennis et al. (eds.), *Contemplating the Role of an Intensive Care Doctor*,
https://doi.org/10.1007/978-3-031-92766-9_15

Consider Your Capacity

When I first became an Attending, I felt like I had to do it all. In order to really prove that I am supposed to be here, I had to do it all. I think that was initially how I felt, and how I thought: "I have to make sure that every patient is okay and like I'm up at night thinking about every patient, what am I doing wrong? Is there something that I'm missing? Oh gosh, what is someone else going to say about my management…" There is a lot of external judgement… a lot of that that you're worried about; and you're like, "What would someone else have done differently"? You know, there's all this stuff that you think about. And then on top of it, "How do I make this other part of my career continue down the path I want it to"? It becomes overwhelming. I think even as an Attending, especially early on, you have to find yourself. It's starting all over again. You have to learn how to be an Attending. When you start, you are going to feel like you are tired all the time; make sure that you spend time; make sure that you do not overextend yourself; don't work on the weekends if you don't have to; try not to do that if you can help it. There are weeks that that's gonna happen; and there's nothing you can do about it but really just make sure you don't lose sight of what's most important. And I think sometimes we feel like this is the most important, and yeah, taking care of patients is important, saving patients is important, but you can't save patients if you can't save yourself.

- It is entirely appropriate to feel like you have limited capacity, but do you regularly explicitly consider and review your capacity?
- Are there any professional roles you might consider relinquishing or putting on hold during particularly busy times, and have you planned and communicated this to the appropriate stakeholders ahead of time?
- Have you considered if and how this might be viewed by others—your reputation?
- Have you thought about your response to these judgements?
- Reflect on the first statement …. 'I felt I had to do it all'. And the last … 'but you can't save patients if you can't save yourself'. Consider what has been modelled for you during your training and what has had the biggest impact on your current work ethic and beyond. Understanding what needs to be done to 'save yourself' is the first step. How easy or hard would it be for you to implement measures that would alleviate or critique the 'do it all' inner voice?
- Who could you talk to about this thought that feels like a conflict, of the pressure of having to do it all on the one hand, yet also having to save yourself first?

Coping with Death

I think the question is, when you have a death, are you going to be the doctor who is completely detached and therefore it doesn't affect you personally, and you can just go on… Somebody died, you know… It's part of the job and you're

alive… It doesn't affect you, right? You don't bring it home. The downside to that though, while that's okay maybe from a personal standpoint, is (whether) that person (is) able to learn from that mistake so that it doesn't happen again with the next patient… Or you have somebody who… on the flipside, if you are very emotionally attached and bring everything home, then it's going to potentially make you into a… your burnout will be very quick, and it may not be good for your mental health. We know, the data shows that acute care providers, whether it is ER, ICU, surgeons… They are the highest risk for divorce; they are the highest risk of suicide; they are the highest risk for substance abuse….

- Death in the ICU is inevitable at some point. Think about a patient death you have experienced that affected you negatively. Can you identify what it was about that death that caused you to have these feelings?
- Is there anything you did when a subsequent patient died to mitigate these things?
- Think about some personal goals to have for yourself in dealing with an unexpected death.
- There may be cumulative effects from working in this setting for a while having to cope with death repeatedly, and this will need some processing even when you think you are coping okay—have you considered setting aside time to do this on a regular basis?
- Processing death takes many forms and varies for individuals—do you know any that works for you? Would you feel safe from negative judgement, discussing this as an ongoing professional development need with your workplace with your line manager?
- Do you believe that spirituality plays a part in your life especially to help you cope with the deaths of your patients? Would you feel safe and comfortable raising this with any of your supervisors, peers where you currently work?
- We all have personal histories and experiences with death too, so how do you take care of yourself when a patient death is especially close to home? Have you prepared yourself for this scenario?

Personal Needs

Well, you feel intensely unhappy. And you sort of want to talk about it, but not talk about it. You don't want people to just tiptoe around you and stuff like that, you want to be supported but not denying. So, people, just being present, supportive, but not pretending. At the same time not prodding, prodding, prodding. You need reassurance. You need some company otherwise you sort of wallow in your own thoughts. You need a little distraction to stop you from doing that as well. So, you need people to distract you, as well. So, they're the things… otherwise… you ruminate... You overly ruminate on these things. When what you really need is distraction, or it's perhaps someone just to talk to frankly….

- Imagine that you have been part of an episode of patient care within your ICU where the outcome was unpredictably poor. Consider how, when and with whom you will evaluate the episode?
- Consider what you might need from those around you at work and what role they would play in your processing of the event.
- Consider what you might need from those around you at home and what role they would play in your processing of the event.
- Have you had this discussion with these people already, and do they understand what you might need from them, and how they could best help in that situation?
- If you have already experienced an event like this, what worked well for you, and what didn't? Is there anything you might change moving forward?
- Have you received any teaching or supervision to specifically help you with this myriad of feelings and the possible range of reactions …from 'distraction' to 'someone just to talk to frankly'?
- What does 'being present' mean to you?
- Your needs for support may vary depending on the circumstances of an incident which is causing you to 'feel intensely unhappy'. You might need different people at different times both at work and in your personal life to support you. Do you have this range of support, and how might you reach out to create this for yourself?

Time-Out

"Make sure you spend time for you and it's okay", we are all in our career, most of the time, we are overachievers. And we want to do things for a multitude of reasons, most importantly we are trying to improve care. Meaning we want to fix people; we're fixers. And when we try to fix people, we forget about ourselves, and we lose sight of important aspects of life. And that is nothing about work-life balance, it's blending that life and understanding that there are going to be weeks that are going to be harder than others; but when you feel yourself getting to the edge of your capabilities, your bandwidth is stretched, stop! And recognise that. And it doesn't mean that you are weak. It doesn't mean that you can't do it, it means that you choose to put you first or your family first as a priority.

I think I went through a period of my life where I just did shift work and stopped playing sports and justified that it was too hard to do a lot of things that aren't work. And I would tell myself not to let that happen again. I think I've got that back.

- Many trainees find the demands of the job to be all-consuming and, as a result, may withdraw from other aspects of their life that might have been helpful to their overall well-being. What specific things are you going to continue to do or start doing for yourself during training?

- Is there anything you have stopped doing that upon reflection might help you now to disconnect from the workplace and provide some balance?
- When you find yourself thinking … 'it's too hard when it is not work', how might you come back from that? What reminders might you need to come back from that position?
- What are your early warning signs that you are overstretching yourself so that you can pull back or get help to pull back?
- Would it be easier to structure 'non-negotiables' that you like doing for yourself no matter the work pressure? What will stop you from doing that if you think that would be a great strategy?
- If you continued to self-sacrifice without your own time-out to enjoy the things you like doing, what might be the consequences?
- We grow up in families that also model work ethic, and you might have seen self-sacrifice at close range or in your supervisors and colleagues—what do you think the effect of this sort of influence might be on you in shaping your work ethic and inadvertently taken on self-sacrifice without being aware of it?
- Does your workplace culture reward a work ethic of self-sacrifice and therefore create a culture of unsustainable work practices? What have you observed so far in your workplace or in your training programme?

Consider Mistakes

We're all human and I think, as I say to people. You do the ward round and I say, "I know that in the last 24 hours I have made about 5 to 10 mistakes". You just haven't picked them. But I have, I know I have. I can sit here and torture myself over them, I will try to do better next time, and I hope I will fail better. But that's what's going to happen.

- No one wants to make mistakes in medicine, especially within a high-acuity high-stakes area like intensive care medicine, but they do happen. During your working career so far, think about a practical mistake you have made. How did it make you feel and what did you physically do in response?
- What did you or can you take away from the way you processed that event? That is, what was helpful, what would you do differently next time?
- Think about making a clinical mistake within the ICU. What things do you think might mitigate mistake-making for you?
- 'I can sit here and torture myself over them…' is a common reaction to mistakes and trying hard not to repeat any or make any more mistakes but also accepting that it will happen again. What would help you process mistakes in the workplace and at home?
- Self-blame for mistakes can feel tortuous, and mistakes with patient care may happen at any time to any of us. How comfortable would you feel about sharing the mistakes you have made that no one else has picked up but your conscience won't leave you alone, hence the torturous feeling?

- What effect would be sharing your mistakes that no one has picked up on your career? Yet how could you manage this private torture if you did not share it and get help to both process and hopefully prevent future mistakes?
- ICU is a complex system, and mistakes will be occurring within this context; how would a systemic view of mistakes help you feel at a personal level about your sense of your own responsibility for the mistake?

Looking Forward

Sometimes they (trainees) come to me, and they're upset about something… and I tell them two things. I'm like, "You should be upset, because if you're not, then something is not right, and you should find a different job, because these are people's kids". It's good to be upset, but in a productive kind of way, not upset to where it's just making you paralysed, and you are just kind of crying all the time. That's not productive. Being a little bit upset about it is important because that's what makes you better. And it makes you learn, and it shows that you care about what you do. These are not…it's not like you've got the answer of a test wrong; these are somebody's kids. You should be upset; so, I tell them that there's nothing wrong with being upset. But I also try to tell them that they want to try and channel that in a more productive way, and not just be so devastated that they start second-guessing themselves all the time—because that can happen—or (that) they just are paralysed and can't act. So, I will usually also try to tell them that you can only make the best decision that you can with the information available at that time, in real-time. You can't look back and say, "What if", you only had that much information and that's what you've got to work with. It's like what they say… they say medicine is practiced prospectively and you learn it retrospectively. I think that's actually true—you look back at things and that helps you learn, but unfortunately when you practice, you are practising forward with information that's available at a particular point in time. It may be all of it; it may be that you are missing crucial information; you may have some misinformation; but that's what you got, so….

- This quote normalises acceptance of the fact that the ICU is a highly emotive environment where staff will at times be challenged and upset. Have you considered that you might become upset at times while working within the ICU?
- Do you often look back at an event and consider what might have been rather than what occurred? If so, how is that helpful for you to process an event?
- Have you considered the responsibility you might bear as team leader in the ICU? How does it make you feel?
- 'Medicine is practiced prospectively, and you learn it retrospectively …'. How does this statement make you feel about medicine in general and ICU in particular? Is it something you would consider helpful to reflect more on and share in a discussion with others?

- Are there the time and opportunity to pause and reflect on the best course of action in your workplace, or is it so busy this is hardly possible?
- 'It's good to be upset but in a productive way …'. What might this comment mean for you? Can you be upset in front of grieving, distressed devastated families even when you know it is acceptable, 'good' even, and if you aren't that sort of person who will react openly that way, do you feel judged for this? Do you judge yourself for this?
- Who has modelled the best coping strategy for you so far? And why did you find yourself resonating with that person's way of coping, thinking and reacting to feeling upset in the workplace?

Difficulties Over the Life of Your Career

The "trainee in difficulty"…. it's not necessarily translated to the "Consultant in difficulty". It's very much seen as a training thing. It's always sort of wrangled with me because I don't think that that framework for thinking about how to approach trainees in difficulty recognises enough the very factors why they might be in difficulty. (Rather) it's got that resilience, victim-blaming, problem attached to it.

I think everybody cyclically goes through phases of detachment… I think that work stressors play a role in that, as do other stressors….

- As you reflect on these quotes, consider your journey so far and where you currently are in terms of the trajectory of your working life in the intensive care. Can you recognise a time when you experienced personal difficulty in the workplace?
- Think about your personal behaviours and emotions during that time. What did you find useful in propelling yourself forward to a better place?
- What did you find that kept you from moving to a more positive mindset?
- What will you do the next time you begin to experience personal difficulty?
- All of us can get into difficulty over the life of our careers, and the framework this quote refers to implies limitations and a sense of frustration with this framework. What frameworks are you aware of that could assist you in thinking about difficulties in your career so far?
- Consultants and heads of department may also get into difficulty in their careers; what is your experience so far of witnessing this and what happened to them?
- Are there some early warning signs yourself or a colleague may be in difficulty, and how might you respond to this if you notice it in a colleague? How might your workplace respond?

Responsibility

Responsibility is not a backbreaking thing… Like being responsible for something even if it was bad, doesn't have to destroy you; it's good… I think it's good to have an emotional response. It's good to be connected to humanity and be sad when sad things happen; and it's good to figure out if you are responsible for something, and to own that responsibility, that's an empowering thing. Even if it doesn't… Even if it's really sad and depressing….

- Think about your relationship with 'responsibility' in the context of your working life within the intensive care domain. Consider when you might see it as a positive thing and when it is a burden. What does considering 'responsibility' as an empowering thing feel like?
- What does considering 'responsibility' as a discouraging and potentially burdensome thing feel like?
- Sometimes responsibility does feel burdensome and sad and depressing, but how do you stop that feeling from destroying you? How would you discuss this further to help yourself and others grapple with it?

Choose Your Role Models; Choose Your Confidante

Look for someone to learn from, but also to learn from everyone. Some people have bad attributes, that it's good to see how you wouldn't want to handle things certain ways.

I would choose who I debriefed to, and… learn who those people are from experience… people with a bit of wisdom, who will give you a fair hearing, who aren't going to be too critical. Like some people who work in ICU are very clever, but sometimes I feel like they can't identify with the common man… people like that are early in their career, they can be a little, or very critical, and [they] just can't understand that perfect medicine doesn't exist….

- Most people want honest feedback on performance - particularly when things don't go as planned—because learning from misadventure is an enormous mitigator of distress. Choosing the best person to deliver that feedback is an important piece of growing personal resilience. Think of a time when you debriefed to someone, and it made you feel worse. Why was that?
- Think of a time when you debriefed to someone, and it made a real positive difference to the way you felt. Why was that?
- If you made an important clinical error today in the management of a patient, think of the things you would need to hear from the person you chose to informally debrief to?

- If you made an important clinical error today in the management of a patient, think of who you would choose to informally debrief to? There may be more than one person—each for different elements.

Litigation

They couldn't find anyone as an expert to say I did anything wrong… but it took five years. So, for seven years… Like the day you get sued, you're like "Oh… crap"! And then nothing happened for a year or two… So you sort of just, move on… being very practical… I guess for me it was a practical survival. Just move on and learn. But it's strange because you can't really share much until after [the case] is closed.

- Across medicine, the threat of litigation is ever-present. This is especially evident within the intensive care setting, where there is high acuity and often a high level of emotional distress. There is often an extended timeframe for resolution of litigation, and this may be to the detriment of the healthcare provider at the centre of the case. Imagine you were recently involved in an important clinical error related to the management of a patient and were informed that the patient had initiated legal action against you. Consider how you will manage your feelings related to this. Who will you tell?
- How will you feel when you hear that there are doctors from other institutions who have been called to testify in the case?
- It could also take a long time before such cases are resolved, and it is crucial that you have support around you during this time, which could be extended. Information and knowledge are other sources of support which you might ask for from your indemnity lawyers who have experience in similar cases and can offer a great deal of advice. It can be very stressful to be sued, and the uncertainty of when there will be an outcome can add to that stress, so it is important to gain perspective from trusted sources which may not be your friends or family who will be anxious and scared on your behalf.
- Do you have private indemnity insurance even during your training, as most hospitals have limited medicolegal support to offer you. Especially in view of the timeframe for some cases to settle, you may have left the workplace where the incident happened; it is important to ensure you have adequate insurance cover.
- The isolation of being sued … 'can't really share much until the case is closed' … is again very good reason to have private indemnity insurance cover as they will be your team to share with and draw support from as well. Being practical and moving on are very good advices in these instances, and how would you do this for yourself?
- Who can you recruit to help you to stay practical and hopeful during this difficult time?

- Litigation cases and outcomes may also get published in the media—do you
  know of any such cases where you work? How can this subject be further discussed in your professional setting? Doctors are not trained to deal with these
  situations or to give evidence, and this may be a subject for professional development for your workplace to consider or talks from doctors with lived experience
  of being sued may be of practical assistance.

Satisfaction

**Where when the outcome is clearly going to be something bad, you can help. I
take great professional satisfaction in this. When you know that the outcome is
going to be bad, you can help the family retain a degree of dignity and allow
that process to unfold in a way that is as respectful to the families as possible.
A way that allows them to dictate what happens as much as possible, that years
down the road, they can look back and say, "If this was going to have to happen, I would have wanted to make sure that we did A, B and C", and to be able
to facilitate that, and sort of allow the death to be as dignified as possible.**

- Rescuing a patient is clearly a rewarding experience, but have you contemplated
  the reward in providing a pathway towards the patient experiencing a dignified death?
- Palliative care physicians specialise in providing patients with as dignified a
  death as possible. If you have not had this experience yourself nor observed your
  supervisors, then it could be something to ask for proactively—input or instruction as to how you could learn to do this more effectively in the ICU setting.
- The dignified death is also a comfort for the families—have you considered how
  this could be facilitated in your ICU setting? There is much to be said for adequate preparation to facilitate a dignified death and rather than learning in retro-
  spect as the quote suggests. What can you learn proactively, and who can you ask
  to do this for yourself and for your ICU if it isn't already in place?
- Asking for support from other colleagues in different specialities may seem
  unusual—or not—depending on your workplace, and it models how, as individual doctors, we may also ask for outside help at our workplaces.

Intensive Care Is a Team Sport

**I can definitely say at the time, "You know this patient would have died if it
wasn't for what we do" and the other thing I feel like I believe, about my role
as an Attending right now, I don't take things on as my... I don't feel at all like
I work in a vacuum. I really believe... when it comes to successes, for sure I
don't work in a vacuum. So, if I believe that's true for success, I also have to**

believe that's true at some level (for lack of success) … And that helps me a lot when things go wrong.

- Teamwork is such an important aspect of ICU care. As someone who may often function in a team leader role, sometimes the responsibility of leadership eclipses the value of teamwork. On reflection, do you often only consider your own role within a challenging patient-care event, or do you also consider how well team members contributed.
- Do you think that the way the team works is always a reflection of the leadership?
- Think of a time when as an individual you privately celebrated the success of your team in managing a challenging patient-care event. Was that easy to recollect?
- Think of a time when as an individual you privately lamented the failure of the team in managing a challenging patient-care event. Was that easy to recollect? Is it easy to recollect the gaps that occurred in the team, or is it easier to recount your own failings during that event?
- Is the teamwork concept embedded and recognised on a regular basis regardless of outcome at your place of work, or is it an assumption that is celebrated usually when there is a positive outcome? How might being recognised as a team on a regular basis in an intentional manner be helpful for the work? How could you lead this as a member of the ICU team where you work?
- Are there other sources of information and inspiration for teamwork and recognition as a team that you could draw from such as from sports clubs or similar organisations outside of medicine?

Conclusion

There is an endless amount of information about self-care and related themes about resilience on the Internet now as compared to when I was a junior doctor, but the universality of doctors having to cope with—and evolve from—witnessing pain and suffering in their patients and containing the levels of distress has not changed over the history of the medicine and related allied health fields. If anything, the widespread availability of information has made it more confusing to access help for ourselves either proactively or reactively, and there is perhaps the additional burden of the expectation of being organised about self-care. Self-care is not always self-evident, and the pathways to accessing help are not always obvious either. There is also the personal risk of exposure and associated vulnerability for those asking for help or admitting to not coping that contributes to the stigma of help-seeking, further compounding the issues faced by doctors working in high-risk areas such as the ICU setting.

Hospitals as employers have increasingly outsourced assistance for doctors to Human Resources (HR) and other management structures or to external psychological agencies to assist doctors in distress, but it is imperative that medicine remembers how to look after its very own—the medical practitioners. Whilst non-medical staff are competent and highly skilled in how their processes and skills can be of assistance, it is my belief and professional experience of years of working with doctors and medical students that the unique set of challenges for the doctor almost always will also require the input, guidance of another doctor colleague or confidante to fully appreciate and process, together, in order to optimise the helping experience for the doctor.

I hope this chapter will stimulate more discussion and generate more contemporary ideas on how hospital systems may consider introducing structured supervision and other specific training on this important topic of self-care in the context of caring for others.

Chapter 16
When Ropes Get Tangled: Contemplating Change

Luke Torre and Andrew Holt

It is not the strongest of the species that survives, nor the most intelligent that survives. It is the one that is most adaptable to change.
– Charles Darwin

The glory of God is a human fully alive.
– Irenaeus

A complex career comes with many challenges. It is self-evident that life is complicated; the path trod by each of us is different and unique. Doctors are not immune to life's everyday challenges: illness, love, children, aging, caring for parents, managing relationships, dealing with loss, finding meaning, and the list is endless. Compound that with the challenges of a trainee and specialist in intensive care, and it is clearly not a career for the faint-hearted.

Intensive care is the specialty of specialties. It houses the doctors on whom other doctors call for help when there is a crisis. It is a high-stakes game, death is common, decisiveness is required, and order must be made from chaos to give the best chance of a positive patient outcome, whether that be returning home alive and well or dying peacefully, surrounded by loved ones.

When can it go wrong in a professional sense? What ropes can get tangled? What missteps on that career tightrope does an intensivist face, and how can they be ameliorated? We have explored some of these questions within the book already. The following chapter considers our career as intensivists longitudinally, as we discuss the stress of questioning career choices, issues around aging gracefully, having it all, and seeing the wood for the trees.

L. Torre (✉)
Department of Intensive Care, Sir Charles Gairdner Hospital, Perth, Australia
e-mail: luke.torre@health.wa.gov.au

A. Holt
Esplanade, Brighton, South Australia, Australia

© The Author(s), under exclusive license to Springer Nature
Switzerland AG 2025
D. Dennis et al. (eds.), *Contemplating the Role of an Intensive Care Doctor*,
https://doi.org/10.1007/978-3-031-92766-9_16

Questioning Career Choices

I go through phases of questioning my career. I presume everybody does… not everybody, but most people do… I can't imagine everybody on the planet is, you know… born a colorectal surgeon and remains that way until they die. To the point where I've made significant enquiries into abandoning medicine, within the last 10 years….

As one progresses through their development in the intensive care specialty, there are a myriad of things to generate stress in any individual. One of these triggers for more senior trainees and junior consultants is reduced training or practice opportunities, with the presumption that they are already adequately trained and practiced. While this has clear patient safety issues, actual or perceived lack of training can also adversely affect confidence and ability to care for critically ill patients. These feelings may contribute to an individual's wellness and enjoyment of work, leading them to question their career decision. This can be amplified in an environment where everyone else appears to be coping, such that it may be difficult to seek help or talk about your inner fears and questions.

Intensive care patients have increasing complexity covering the entirety of acute medicine, and there may also be fewer teaching opportunities given the overall level of patient acuity. Reduced anaesthesia training time, for example, which directly affects critical airway skills, is likely to add to the stress of the senior trainee rostered out of hours. We have heard anecdotally that some senior Australian trainees undertake less than ten intubations per year. A small number of highly technical time-critical procedures are required to be mastered, and competition for learning opportunities (for both consultant and trainee doctors) relating to these 'top end' procedures can be unhealthy. It may be that a more rigorous determination of 'Scope of Practice' is needed for our specialty to ensure safe practice and positive well-being.

There may also be reduced training opportunities associated with the increasing numbers of trainees and thereby reduced intensive care patient exposure. This is compounded by the rostering of trainees to alternate responsibilities, such as Medical Emergency Teams, teaching and research duties, and ward outreach activities (e.g. parenteral nutrition and tracheostomy management).

Lack of training or practice opportunity is just one example of something that might elicit negative thoughts or questions about career choices. There are also other challenges facing trainees that have emerged over the years. For example, there may be an overall heightened sense of responsibility for patient care and outcomes within the intensive care setting, which, although unrealistic, may be nonetheless burdensome. What is important to remember is that, as the quote suggests, most of us will experience these feelings of uncertainty in career choice at one time or other during the span of our working life. During these times, self-reflection is an important process to consider the source of these sentiments and to weigh up the options for response. This is where an individual needs to consider developing their own set of 'Safety Nets'. What that looks like, and how they are defined and established, is discussed in Chap. 17.

Aging Gracefully

I think that for me, the things that would help me best in terms of staying in this career… because like I said I still love what I do. I would like to see myself do less night call. It gets harder and harder to recover from a long night on call. It's harder now than it was 20 years ago, and I think getting older is part of that. I happen to really like mentoring trainees and junior faculty in developing research careers, or research components of their careers and I have been fairly successful in my own research career. So would I like to be able to spend more of my time focusing on that, and less time doing the clinical stuff? Yes. I don't know that there is a percentage… But certainly less night call would allow me to do that without having to go home… The other day I went home after a night on call, and it wasn't a bad night on call but I didn't get a lot of sleep, and I spent eight hours in front of my computer writing a book chapter that was due, as opposed to going home and getting some sleep, or going to the gym - both of which would probably have been better for my physical and mental well-being than sitting in front of the computer. And it's taken until today to just sort of recoup from that, in terms of just feeling less fatigued, and I'm going into another night call.

Aging gracefully within this specialty may be challenging—to expound upon our analogy, the ropes of the most experienced trapeze artist may indeed become tangled, worn, or frayed. The most important thing is to behave in an open and honest way. Dr Andrew Holt describes below how he managed his transition from Critical Care Director to retirement, which was expedited following his diagnosis of Parkinson's disease at the age of 61:

I cannot believe it!! I always thought I would retire on my own terms, how wrong did this prove to be.

I had been proactive in organising the monitoring of my clinical performance by senior colleagues. In addition, I self-amended my scope of practice within the intensive care unit and later the entire hospital. This began initially with cessation of rostering on at intensive care units in the private hospital sector. I remained working within the public sector, where there was readily available backup if required (although during this period I never required backup or intervention in a time critical event).

I next ceased afterhours on-call work, as I recognised my increasing tiredness after a busy on-call shift, whether it was sleep interruption due to multiple phone calls or there was an event which required urgent attendance which involved getting up out of bed and driving quickly and safely to the hospital.

I ceased all ICU procedures, although there had not been any adverse events relating to my procedures, but once again, it was consistent with my approach over this period of being proactive, 'staying in front'. There were some procedures, for example, percutaneous tracheostomy and Hickman catheter insertion, for which I remained a recognised expert by my colleagues. Despite this, an excessive focus on procedures for the elderly ICU specialist prevails.

I was fortunate that part of my original practice was essentially a clinic-based outpatient service for a Home Parenteral Nutrition (PN) Unit. My original 'job plan' was 0.4 full time equivalent (FTE) Home PN and 0.5 FTE ICU. This enabled a change in my scope of practice to Home PN and teaching only which, once again, was self-amended. Being able to slowly contract my practice from ICU to Home PN was considered a good way to proceed. This was considered less of a stress for me; however I'm not sure I completely agreed with this. The patients requiring Home PN were very complex, demanding patients referred state-wide with intestinal failure, and it was my responsibility to manage them. The stress associated with Home PN in fact came more from lack of adequate funding as much as anything. There was also a significant on-call roster commitment, but the requirement for after-hours work was infrequent. My overall belief was that through open discussion, proactive amending of credentialing, and recognised expertise in Home PN and ICU teaching, I had kept well ahead of any concerns relating to my clinical ability.

Six years into a progressive chronic neuro-degenerative disease, as well as managing several other age-related disorders, have I effectively confronted my aging and illness gracefully? Was I safe working within my new job plan? Did my colleagues have confidence in me? Up until this point, I would say 'yes'.

Some elective surgery subsequently hastened my retirement from the specialty I worked in for more than 40 years. Although unpalatable, and incredibly disappointing, it has made me reflect on the fact that it is not necessarily easy to age gracefully within and from the high-pressured environment of an ICU. When time away is needed to attend to your own medical or surgical diagnoses, take more time than you need, and completely sever your personal illnesses from your workplace. Seek help from professionals outside your institution and keep your progress private. Above all, come back when you are fully recovered and ready to go, not before. Do not try to keep doing bits and pieces here and there, or 'help out' when you can, when you are not ready.

What I have learned is the importance of loyalty, the value of insight, and the trust we all need to have in our colleagues both that they can be appropriately proactive in their own practice and can function as a safety net for one other.

Having It All

…I had to normalise the situation because I thought, "I'm failing this; I'm a failure" and so talking with her and hearing someone who was successful say that they had had these same thoughts, it helped. It helped to say this isn't new, this isn't just you, we all go through this. And how do you deal with it? It's making sure that you are not overextending yourself and recognising that that does not mean you are a failure. And I think that's how our society makes you feel sometimes when you are trying to be career oriented and you're trying to have upward mobility within career. Is that if you can't maintain it all, then you've failed a little bit.

I once had an accomplished young female ICU specialist come into my office, sit down, and say, 'I just wish someone had told me years ago… "you can't have it all"'. She was in the middle of arguably the busiest time of her life: a wife, a mother of three young children, a competent full-time ICU specialist, a daughter to elderly frail parents, a sister, an educator, a supervisor of training, a friend. It dawned on her that when all this is happening, it becomes impossible to maintain the high standards you would like across all responsibilities. Something has to give or the ropes start to fray. I think many of us feel like this; I know I do. How we deal with this, if and when it happens, is the challenge.

Ultimately, if we are led by our pride, we will use bad coping mechanisms. We will push on, deny we can't handle it, compartmentalise our lives, wait for something or someone else to crack, strain our relationships, and strain our emotions and our mental health. Yet this seems to be the path most trod.

We need to surrender to humility. To take stock of our priorities, reorder them and rationalise our lives. We must talk to those who are affected, listen, and act. We must acknowledge how we are changing, recognise what we don't like, and commit to rectifying it, whatever the cost.

Seeing the Wood for the Trees

There is a little bit of change in the way ICU is now, relative to what it was when I started. Partially I think because we've gotten so much better at supporting things. We can keep things going for a much longer period of time, without necessarily at this point in time, still having the technology to be able to actually get someone in a better situation. So, you can support much longer than what you can actually cure, per se….

Australian rules football (AFL) is a complex game. Thirty-six players on the field, full contact, and high intensity mean it's easy to focus on simply getting the ball to the immediate next player to not lose possession; possession is key. Far more challenging is the ability to 'lift your eyes' amidst the pressure and chaos and see what is happening further up the field and what longer and better options are on offer if you have the courage, composure, and skill to take them on. They are higher risk, but higher reward and how memorable goals are scored.

In intensive care, it is natural to focus on fixing problems. Every day we make hundreds of decisions designed to manage defined issues. We prescribe dialysis to manage renal failure, analgesics for pain, antibiotics for infection, anti-arrhythmics for atrial fibrillation, heparin for DVT prophylaxis…; the list is endless. We have taken our patient, the human being in front of us, and dismantled them to an abstract set of diagnoses and problems to treat. We reassemble them as organ failures, as electrolyte abnormalities, as symptoms, and as risk factors and prescribe remedies for each. We are truly masters of this and our results are nothing short of miraculous. Our staffing levels, rostering, technologies, and machines have made us indefatigable. We can do this better than ever before, and we can do this forever.

What is far more challenging is to put that aside and 'lift our eyes' to the bigger question of the whole patient outcome. What will happen to this patient in the longer term? What is the pathway from here forward, out of ICU? Can I get this patient home and well? Am I consigning them to a nursing home or a protracted death in hospital? Surely these are the outcomes we need to focus on, not fixing itemised problems. Rather than keeping possession of the football by endlessly solving problems, we need to kick a memorable goal by achieving the best patient outcome.

Often, we refuse to engage with these questions because of the probability problem. We are rarely 100% certain of a patient's outcome, so do we have the right to recommend stopping treatment without the absolute certainty of a bad outcome? Some argue no, which is fair, but the reverse question is just as valid. In patients with a bleak prognosis, do we have the right to continue and create many bad outcomes for real patients (who then must live like this), to justify the potential good outcome that might unexpectedly occur in one? Some of these ethical dilemmas have been discussed already in Chap. 4.

The overarching consensus is that we should think more about our patient as a whole person. We must understand their values and wishes, what 'quality of life' means to them. Have we taken the time to comprehend the life they have led, their life in the present, and the life that lies ahead. We need to be more cognoscente of 'meaning' rather than existence.

The best intensive care doctors are those who can engage with these questions and come to true shared decision-making. This is not paternalism or biased medicine as often claimed. Rather, instead of avoiding the ethical dilemmas of intensive care, these clinicians meet these questions head on. They lift their eyes to the bigger picture and recommend a definitive and courageous path. This is a hallmark of true empathy, clinical acumen, and patient-centred care.

Conclusion

So where have we come from and where are we going? This existential question can and should be applied to our speciality to better understand ourselves. Intensive care was born out of an 'extended recovery room' for patients undergoing major or emergency surgeries unable to go directly to usual hospital wards. It was started by anaesthetists who had an interest in the post-operative care of these patients and the continued use of their interventions like ventilation, vasopressors, pain therapies, and invasive lines. It was straightforward; the support and monitoring devices were limited in type and options; the goals obvious; the medicine completely digestible in books like 'internal medicine'.

Modern intensive care is radically different. Patients have increased complexity covering the entirety of acute medicine. There is no tome that can encompass all medical knowledge, it has exceeded our grasp, and we are doomed to the world of specialists and super-specialists to keep up. The 'single organ doctor' (or SOD) has emerged with all their pros and cons. It has made greater the need for the general knowledge and holistic pragmatism of the intensive care specialist. However, it has made the need to engage with the SOD paramount, firstly, to comprehend their high-end esoteric knowledge and recommendation on the management of the focused problem and, secondly, to relay our holistic view of the long-term trajectory and likely outcome of the actual whole patient.

There is heightened responsibility for patient care and outcome, with ever-increasing expectations of patient, family, and society. Autonomy has improperly become the absolute ethical value. Doctors are considered more like waiters at a restaurant, offering a menu of choices, with no specific recommendation unless asked, waiting to accept the order of the patient and execute it promptly.

Medical rather than surgical diagnoses now comprise an ever-increasing percentage of our cohort. There are fewer quick fixes, more long stay patients, more chronicity, more elderly, and more difficult decisions. There are highly technical, time-critical procedures to be mastered. Devices are becoming more complex and compact, making them more useful and ubiquitous in intensive care. There are more options, brands, modes, and more minimally invasive methods. There is more to know, with potentially less experience. All this suggests patients will continue to have more and more interventions offered, despite increasing age, frailty, and complexity. These are daunting thoughts and mean intensive care needs to function as a collective of expertise and thought and collaborate more with our colleagues to make informed choices.

The whole concept of the physical intensive care unit has also radically changed. It is now a world without borders; the walls have been knocked down. We exist in the realms of rapid response teams, outreach ward rounds, and parenteral nutrition, both inpatient and home based. We follow up patients we have tracheostomised after they leave ICU, and we pre-operatively consult on patient suitability for major surgery. We have long championed the idea of 'goals of care' meetings with patients on admission to hospital, not once they are critically unwell and on machines. We even do longer-term ICU follow-up outpatient clinics! The generalist breadth of the intensivist may add value in all hospital settings. We have a contribution to give most patients, if asked, and offer a valuable perspective often lost in the disease-focused world of hospital medicine. It is likely our roles will extend upwards in the future to executive leadership positions, where we can effectively mediate the competing needs of individual specialties and groups. Our team-based approach and natural leadership skills should make us excellent candidates for these roles.

What does this mean for you, the individual? Far less than you think. The path to a successful career lies hand in hand with the path to a meaningful life. But they are not a linear relationship. The prized title of 'world renowned intensivist' most likely comes at such a significant cost to all other aspects of life, that true meaning and happiness may be lost. It is well-recognised event, when in excitement a doctor meets the child of an esteemed colleague and promptly rushes over to tell them 'Your father/mother is an exceptional doctor'. The reply from the less than impressed child often leaves them shocked 'Yes, I know, shame they aren't an exceptional father/mother'. How do we strike this balance? We must first ask what we want in life and what a life well-lived would look like in 10, 20, 40, and 60 years' time. We must be honest about the answers, and they must be our own, influenced only by our spouse and closest loved ones. Then we can make an initial plan how to get there, a plan that will undergo countless revisions, but under the same rubric.

In the desert, Christ was tempted three times by Satan. Those temptations were themed around power, pleasure, and pride. A meaningful career must be one where these are resisted at every turn. It is doubtless these temptations will come; it is how we respond to them that will define our happiness.

We must also remember how privileged we are to be intensive care doctors. We will all save countless lives, cure disease, prevent morbidity, and alleviate suffering. Without necessarily being exceptional, we achieve exceptional results every day. We will work in exciting multi-disciplinary team-based environments, meeting and interacting with wonderful people daily. Knowing them better and seeing the person behind the position will add so much to your job satisfaction. Most importantly, we will interact with patients and their families. Those interactions are our career. How you carry out those episodes of care defines who you are as a specialist above all else. You will make a difference every single day; what kind of difference is up to you.

So, when missteps happen, stand tall, look upwards and forwards, balance yourself, and keep walking along the tightrope. You, the trapeze artist, can get to the other side.

Chapter 17
Installing Safety Nets: Contemplating Our Fieldwork Guide

Rakesh Khanna (ID)

> *The sharp edge of a razor is difficult to pass over; thus, the wise say the path to Salvation is hard.*
>
> – *Katha Upanishad*

Intensive care units are one of the most intense and busy areas of any major medical facility. Despite some overt similarities, each person coming to the ICU is a unique individual in a unique set of circumstances. The ICU team also consists of several unique individuals with their own set of knowledge, skills and experience base.

Choosing to work in the intensive care setting is akin to participation in extreme sports. Brain chemistry and hormones may determine why people enjoy the thrill of extreme sports. There is a sense of achievement and pride attached to accomplishing something that normally people are unable to do otherwise. At the same time, there are greater chances of having to face adverse outcomes and the possibility of death. Intensive care workers need to make split-second decisions which are likely to have major consequences, sometimes highly detrimental.

A long-held colloquialism holds that the four ideal attributes of a good surgeon include eagle's eyes, crow's decision, lady's fingers and lion's heart. Working in the ICU requires all these attributes, but they are sufficient only when the situation is unambiguous. Success in ICU is also contingent upon the unit working as a team. It is a real test of the four C's of cognitive science: critical thinking, creativity, communication and collaboration.

From a psychological perspective, there are several important dimensions to working in the ICU. The contemplative parts of the book pointed to the many vulnerability factors of importance in the context of working in the ICU setting. All interactions occur in a certain 'setting' (ICU) and involves 'the individual' (intensive care physician) in relation to 'the others' (members of the team) and in a certain 'context' which includes 'the one in the eye of the storm', 'the carers' and sometimes those 'for whom the bell tolls'. In this chapter we will work on installing

R. Khanna (✉)
Northpark Hospital, Bundoora, VIC, Australia

© The Author(s), under exclusive license to Springer Nature
Switzerland AG 2025
D. Dennis et al. (eds.), *Contemplating the Role of an Intensive Care Doctor*,
https://doi.org/10.1007/978-3-031-92766-9_17

safety nets considering what has been contemplated in the previous sections of the book.

The Setting: ICU Signifies a Spectre of Uncertainty

In Chap. 8 we talked about 'contemplating the place', where the ICU setting was likened to a stormy sea. This is because a lot happens at the same time in the confines of ICU. Patients here are, by their very nature, some of the sickest in the hospital. Clinical algorithms can be useful for run-of-the-mill clinical situations; however, statistics are about averages and not the individual patient being treated. There are many variations in human biology and hence pathology. At any time, intensive care doctors are dealing with individuals rather than an aggregate of humankind.

ICU is also a very dynamic place where priorities change all the time. Behind the veneer of competence and confidence lurk many degrees of uncertainties in the mind of experts [1]. Groopman quoted Jay Katz who examined the defences that physicians deploy against awareness of uncertainty. He first looked at Renny Fox's identification of three basic types of uncertainty: incomplete or imperfect mastery of available knowledge; limitations of current medical knowledge; and difficulty distinguishing between personal ignorance or ineptitude and limitations of current medical knowledge. Katz lumped Fox's three categories together under disregard for uncertainty. He argued that while uncertainty itself poses a significant burden on physicians, the greater burden is the obligation to keep these uncertainties in mind and acknowledge them to patients. The denial of uncertainty—the proclivity to substitute for uncertainty—is one of humanity's most remarkable psychological traits. It is both adaptive and maladaptive, guiding and misguiding physicians alike. Physicians' denial of awareness of uncertainty makes matters seem clearer, more understandable and more certain than they are [2]. Such denial is adaptive. In real time medical practice decisions must be made despite all uncertainties.

Daniel Kahneman [3] suggested: 'Learning medicine consists in part of learning the language of medicine. Systematic errors are known as biases, and they record predictably in particular circumstances. Most impressions and thoughts arise in your conscious experience without your knowing how they got there. The mental work that produces impressions, intuitions, and many decisions go on in silence in your mind. We are often confident even when we are wrong, and an objective observer is more likely to detect our errors than we are'.

None of us are immune to 'cognitive dissonance'. When reality clashes with our deepest convictions, we recalibrate reality rather than amend our world view. A round-the-clock service is associated with the emotions of the various care providers and those of patients and families. One has to deal with a plethora of emotions and interpersonal issues on the run.

The Individual: Intensive Care Physician

Chapter 6 involved 'contemplating your personality'. Interestingly, the word 'personality' did not exist in English until the eighteenth century, and the idea of 'having a good personality' only became widespread in the twentieth century [4]. Susman termed it as it a shift from a 'Culture of Character' to a 'Culture of Personality'[5]. She wrote, 'Every American was to become a performing self'. The focus until then was on character formation. It spread to the rest of the western world and beyond, even though most people lie somewhere on a spectrum of extroversion and introversion.

Personality is 'the dynamic organisation within the individual of those psychophysiological systems that determines his unique adjustment in his environment' [6]. Various combinations of the following five factors of personality define the uniqueness of a person and their particular ways of relating to people and circumstances.

These factors include the following:

1. Neuroticism (a tendency to be depressed, anxious and stress reactive)
2. Agreeableness (an orientation towards empathy and getting along with other people)
3. Extroversion (a disposition to be outgoing, friendly and emotionally positive)
4. Conscientiousness (a tendency to be orderly and achievement oriented)
5. Openness (a tendency to be curious, imaginative and to try new change)

Roles are defined by the training of the person involved. In every multidisciplinary team, there is a need for collaboration and a degree of flexibility in the team to ensure more effective functioning. The role of the intensivist was explored in Chap. 7.

Our biological building block consists of DNA's double helix, but real-life building blocks include physiological, experiential and socio-cultural elements [7]. Vulnerabilities may arise from within us and is also influenced by the social and cultural context in which we are operating. There are general and individual vulnerability factors. People pick careers in medicine with goals such as saving lives. Those choosing intensive care as a career may be keener on being at the forefront of the act of saving lives. Dying is not slow when observed real time. Ernest Becker posits humans use denial to erase death probability such that we do not realise reacting to existential fear [8]. Medicine peels back this layer of denial just enough for conscious awareness. Being a doctor means living with fear incorporated into daily life. Lifton introduced the concept of 'psychological closure' as a distinctive pattern of response to overwhelming threatening stimuli [9]. It is a highly adaptive response and often a means of emotional self-preservation. Eventually, this form of denial gives way, and one is left to deal with the bottled-up emotions.

Every individual has many roles to play. Besides being an intensivist, one is also a person with a personal life. One has to deal with the usual trials and tribulations of life. We learn to try to compartmentalise personal problems when we are at work, but it may not always be quite so easy. We may also be carrying the burden of some of our negative past experiences, both personal and professional.

A medical practitioner's calm stance should appear apparent to patients/families. No one expects infallibility. Medicine remains an uncertain science where do no harm stands paramount. Despite decades' experience fears persist over harming/causing patient death never completely dissipates.

Perfectionism, common among doctors, serves as a double-edged sword—unmet lofty expectations may lead to increased stress/anxiety/depression levels. Empathy involves understanding patient feelings without necessarily experiencing them oneself—a cognition allowing standing in the others' shoes while retaining ones' own position. Some of the challenges to empathy arise from cultural and language barriers. The doctor needs to be able to clearly communicate that understanding [10]. Most patients' anger and resultant lawsuits stem from the doctor's lack of empathy and genuine communication.

The Context: The Other Participants

Working in the ICU invariably involves functioning as part of a team. Interpersonal relationship troubles arise from either intruding on other people's tasks or having one's own tasks intruded upon. Initially, one should inquire whose task it is [12]. Care in the ICU is continuous, with several handovers per day among different combinations of care team members. Healthcare is a collaborative endeavour, and teamwork is particularly crucial in the ICU. No amount of planning can foresee all eventualities.

Chapter 9 was about 'diagnosing bias'. It dealt with the various aspects of clinical practice involving judgement of several types. Perceptions of discrimination and biases are inherent part of everyday life. It can be just more intense in an ICU setting as a result of the sheer pace at which they unfold.

The Context: The One in 'The Eye of The Storm"

Patients come to the ICU either directly via an ambulance through the emergency department or indirectly following transfer from other wards of the hospital. A medical crisis, a call for ambulance, the impatience associated with the time taken for the ambulance to arrive, a quick evaluation and decision to take the patient to ICU/ED with sirens blaring is enough to raise immense anxiety in the patient. This may be the first such experience and therefore even more anxiety-provoking. Most people will never be totally desensitised to it despite repeated visits.

Those transferred from within the hospital would indeed be conscious of their deteriorating medical condition to warrant such transfer. The busy setting of the ICU with the hurried movement of the staff, the beeping of monitors, and all the tubes, wires, and machines is enough to raise alarm signals in even the most stoic. Anxiety can be contagious, and calm heads are needed not only for the most effective care for the patients but also for the patient to feel reassured that they are receiving the best and proper care.

In Chap. 13 the special aspects of pediatric critical care were considered. Children can be more vulnerable to adverse outcomes. Parents and significant others have huge emotional investment in children. They have the task of raising, protecting and advocating for the child. To lose a parent or a lifelong friend is often to lose the past: the person who died may be the only other living witness of golden events of long ago. But, to lose a child is to lose the future: what is lost is no less than one's life project—what one lives for, how one projects oneself into the future and how one may hope to transcend death [11]. Loss of an adult is 'object loss' (the object being a figure who has played an instrumental role in the constitution of one's inner world), whereas child loss is 'project loss' (the loss of one's central organizing life principle, providing not only the why but also the how of life).

The Context: For Whom the Bell Tolls

Most often, a classification of a person's dying is a psychosocial process. Besides objective facts it reflects the background, information needs and motives of person who is making the classification. Because each person has his own framework, it is not surprising the onset of dying process often registers at different points in time in the minds of various people involved [13]. Despite all odds, patients and families may still be hanging on to the hope of a good outcome.

Chapter 11 expounded the need for 'singing from the same songbook'. Managing family dynamics is part of the complexity of working in the ICU, and they may be accentuated in the crisis that people find themselves when confronted with a serious medical condition. Various family members may react differently. The struggle is to keep the trust of the family while being able to support them through the crisis of having to face a serious illness of their family member and then potentially also cope with the grief of a fatal outcome.

It helps to have all members of the ICU healthcare team be unified as conflicting information is likely to create difficulties. It is also important to determine the team member best equipped to deal with the family members. A brief huddle of the team before approaching the family can be particularly important. Chapter 13 describes the experiences of two intensivists who led from the front during the COVID-19 pandemic. Working in ICU during such time was particularly challenging given the paucity of information about the condition and its management. The emotional cost for those involved was palpably very high. In Chaps. 12 and 13, we considered contemplating communication with other doctors and with our own team, and these aspects of honest communication are always critically important.

Installing Safety Nets

Having established the intensity of the ICU setting where one is continuously exposed to a taxing high-octane taking environment, the need for an individual to install appropriate safety nets is self-evident as we can all be vulnerable to some extent and at certain times and circumstances. Every thread, whatever material they are made of, has its breaking point. To survive well and work optimally in what one has chosen to do requires adequate self-care.

We set the scene for this self-care in Chap. 5, where we asked the reader to self-reflect on what first interested them in intensive care and introduced five extremely useful antidotes. We focussed on the shadows of doubt that those working in the ICU face and suggested ways of learning to climb the ropes in Chap. 15. Let's now focus on the individual's safety nets.

The term 'individual' refers to being a single entity that cannot be divided. The individual decides on a life script—an unconscious blueprint for one's life course—which encompasses personality variables and repetitive interpersonal interactions. Life scripts are neither written at one specific time in life nor set in stone; most people continue to revise their life scripts over time. Our life experiences and circumstances are primary motivating factors affecting these changes. Sometimes we do this consciously; at other times, changes occur subtly and imperceptibly.

The self is a mental representation of oneself, representing our knowledge of ourselves. The self consists of stories we tell about ourselves—stories relating to how we got where we are, why we did what we did and what happened next. We rehearse these stories internally to remind ourselves of who we are and share them with others to encourage them to form a particular impression of us. These stories change as our self-understanding or strategic self-representation evolves.

The self is also a bundle of propositions about our abstract traits and specific experiences, thoughts, and actions, where semantic self-knowledge is represented independently of episodic self-knowledge [14]. As the preface of the book very succinctly points out: 'Each of us has a unique set of personal characteristics that define our capability, and we should therefore seek to consider our own bespoke set of solutions to the problems and issues that arise in our life'.

Existential Formulation

A four-dimensional model of existence encompasses: (1) a physiological self, (2) an experiential self, (3) a socio-cultural self, and (4) an existential self. The existential dimension is in effect the art of sense making and stance taking [7].

Addressing Physiology

Our body is the basic unit of our existence. A healthy lifestyle is essential for physiological integrity, including a good diet, regular exercise routine, maintaining a good sleep-wakefulness cycle, and avoiding excesses in everything.

Maintaining a regular schedule is challenging due to human-made light disturbing our sleep-wakefulness cycle along with other biological rhythms. Gadgets like television, computers, Internet access, and smartphones are major distractions.

We are encouraged towards greater achievement and stretching ourselves towards creating a bigger impact on the world stage. When stressed for whatever reasons, two processes occur simultaneously: improving our ability to overcome stressful situations while stress makes us less efficient in doing so. A vicious cycle ensues where all biological rhythms are out of tune.

Stress is a major factor in burnout and has received increasing attention. ICU by its very nature needs to operate round the clock and workforce is essential to its functioning. Staff must work in shifts and hence one has to work harder to maintain our biological rhythms.

Our physiology works on a template formed about 40–50 thousand years ago; however, our current lifestyle vastly differs from those times when physical activity was driven by hunting needs or gathering resources like food or water. Even after transitioning to growing food or managing other necessities, using human power alone was still prevalent until societies became more organised through technology-driven cooperation requiring much less physical effort than ever before.

The long hours of work and changing schedules may make it more likely for the ICU workers to show poor engagement in self-care and failure to follow basic health recommendations. When one suffers from other medical problems, attention is necessary to manage them appropriately.

Stress and feelings have been seen as universally overwhelming, and hence hospitals now hold stress management workshops/support groups/mindfulness meditation sessions as part of prevention plans. However, often people are too busy incorporating another beneficial activity into their daily routine to take advantage of these resources.

Antonio Damasio [15] describes the emotions as the 'continuous musical line of our minds, the unstoppable humming'. Emotions can often be the dominant player in medical decision-making, handily overshadowing evidence-based medicine, clinical algorithms, quality control measures, and even medical experience. And this can occur without anyone's conscious awareness [10].

Addressing Experiential Issues

Our past experiences, particularly traumatic ones, shape us in many ways. Such experiences stay is our memories and can affect us adversely. They can cause physiological arousal and affect emotionally even when they do not constitute a post-traumatic stress disorder (PTSD), whether acute or chronic. Trauma is ubiquitous but humans are resilient, and PTSD is not an invariable consequence. Trauma may have occurred in our personal and family life or working life. When exposed to similar situations again, this is likely to induce an emotional response.

In situations like these, people often seek support informally through colleagues and partners, perceiving that outsiders cannot completely understand the complexity of distress related to ICU work. Exposing emotions in front of colleagues may have deleterious effects if the response is offensive. Time constraints and lack of follow-up are additional problems with this approach. Demonstrating vulnerability may not be appropriate in every work environment and could lead to further emotional distress.

Interpersonal life is all about effective communication. In Chap. 2 we described the two contrasting models: communication as information transfer and communication as social construction. Creating effective information transmission involves understanding and anticipating the information needs and readiness of the receiver. Each discipline has its own language, and it is important to be mindful of how they may affect problems in communication.

Status hierarchy is an inevitable part of any organisation and ICU is no exception. The type of hierarchy may vary with significant implications for its functioning. Susan Cain [3] quotes studies to point out that, contrary to the general belief, the more effective leaders were those with little or no 'charisma'. Such leaders were more interested in listening and gathering information than in asserting their opinion or dominating conversation. Extroverts are often so intent on their own stamp on events that they risk losing others' innovative ideas and allowing workers to lapse into passivity.

From an individual psychological perspective, Adler saw all emotional difficulties as arising from interpersonal difficulties. Interpersonal relations are the source of unhappiness. He advocated for the concept of horizontal relationships [12]. The most important guiding principle is not to judge others. Judgment arises from vertical relationships. In horizontal relationships, words of straightforward gratitude, respect and joy prevail. In group debriefing settings, the intensivist is viewed as the leader. It would be highly unusual for the senior staff to share his emotions effectively in such a forum and benefit emotionally from it.

Addressing Social and Cultural Issues

Humans are biological, psychological, as well as social entities, and the three aspects of their existence are always interacting and influencing each other. Our social and cultural milieu influence us in many ways. Society and culture certainly change over time. There is a macro-culture and a micro-culture, and we usually live in a micro-culture which is more conducive to our healthy living. One can develop a more fulfilling relationship within it.

In the face of an adverse outcome, it is natural to develop a perception of being blamed followed by a sense of humiliation and shame, and their consequences can be devastating. We automatically erect walls to hide it, and they become a major impediment to the full disclosure policies that are increasingly demanded. No matter how rational we claim to be, the fragility of human heart can prevail over data, ethics and even laws.

Clinicians fear causing patient harm and can be gripped by a sense of shame post-critical incident. Acceptance of the inevitability of medical error/patient death mitigates emotional fallout, fostering a realistic work attitude. Even excellent training does not preclude mistakes. When one is doing the wrong thing, it may still feel the same as doing the right thing. One does not know it is wrong or that the act is not going to turn out the way it should have until after it has occurred. Remaining calm, in charge, but open to suggestions from others is a skill that continues to improve throughout one's career.

Legal systems are an integral part of the social and cultural process. Dealing with a lawsuit is often likened to having a death in the family. Unlike other medical settings, in the ICU one does not have the luxury of refraining from taking on patients who are perceived as challenging or who have complicated medical issues. Many doctors feel embittered, having lost the joy of medicine. Every doctor feels their competence and identity as a doctor challenged, even if the suit is entirely frivolous. All sued doctors change how they practise—in ways both large and small—and this can have wide-ranging effects on patients.

Addressing Existential Issues

Humans are complex beings. We not only exist, but we are also conscious of our existence as well as have a concept of non-existence. Our consciousness includes a sense of self and that of other people, other living beings, vegetation, objects and the environment. We develop a narrative of self and our surrounding. We continuously observe through our senses, make mental impressions of what we observe, create images, analyse and interpret them through the passage of life. Our experiences shape us from birth to death, and we also try to imagine what would happen to us beyond death and to those who will survive us. Our conscious experience is to a considerable extent determined by the linguistic concepts we use to understand the world around us.

Coping strategies are thoughts and behaviours used to manage stressful situations. Problem-focused strategies involve acting on the environment to remove the stressors or fix the problem. In interpersonal relationships, focused coping support is sought from people. The usefulness of a particular strategy depends on the person using it and the specific stressors they are experiencing.

I. Cognitive behavioural approach

Thought processes associated with anxiety and depression can be conceptualised as problems of logic. Informal cognitive behavioural approaches have been used by all good parents, teachers, elders of any community and mentors through the ages. It is often said: 'Science is nothing but refined everyday thinking'.

Cognitive behavioural therapy aims to help identify and challenge unhelpful thoughts and to learn practical self-help strategies. These strategies are designed to bring about immediate positive changes in quality of life. It helps us challenge unhelpful thoughts and has been successfully used for a wide range of conditions. Emotions may be even more important determinant of behaviour. Cognition is to a considerable extent also governed by emotions. They are interconnected processes. Being adapt at analysing our cognitions allows us to look at alternative ways of looking at it and in the process find more adaptive ways of functioning.

II. Mindfulness-based approach

Mindfulness is a central theme in Buddhism. There is significant overlap in beliefs held in Buddhism and Stoicism. Epictetus believed: 'People are not disturbed by things but by the view they take on them'. The view taken may, in fact, denote sense-making. Seneca wrote: 'There are more things to alarm us than to harm us, and we suffer more in apprehension than in reality'. Anxiety is apprehension of what could go wrong. Depression and hopelessness are about a loss of a worthwhile future. Managing anxiety involves learning to live better in an unknown future.

Mindfulness-based therapies include the concept of 'the wise mind'. The reasonable mind is about thoughts or cognition, emotional mind signifies affects or emotions, and the wise mind is the joint operation of cognition, emotion and wisdom. Working on specific skills that can help people to be in a wise state of mind can be rewarding. 'We are all imperfect people living in an imperfect world' is a concept that can be used quite broadly and effectively.

III. Sense-making

Insight involves sense-making, and it is usually related to a specific aspect of life and in a particular situation. Existential therapy aims at providing the freedom to maintain a flexible and relative stance. Everyone can take a unique perspective on oneself and one's situation with better outcome.

Existential formulation can be used for 'disease' states (signifying pathology) as well as states of 'dis-ease' (altered states of being with the ability to get back in order, returning to a state of ease). Both disease and dis-ease are likely to be accompanied by perturbations in physiology. Most of those working in ICU are likely to be in dis-ease and not diseased. Admittedly, the distinction may be difficult to determine at times.

'Sense-making' can be defined as a person's evaluative interaction with his/her environment. It is more than a cognitive process. Emotions play an especially important part in our cognitive processes. Part of emotion is conveyed in words or feelings, but some remain at just the visceral level. There is a fundamental interdependence between feelings and thinking in human social life. Our affective experiences are integrally linked with how information about the world is stored. Affect can influence both the process of thinking and the content of thinking. Sense-making can occur in isolation or with mentors, and in Chap. 3 we pointed to a range of positive outcomes associated with mentoring and the vulnerability of self-reflection.

At the heart of an existential mode of thinking is the importance of identifying the 'I' or 'me' as the centre of my universe. This is followed by a sense of freedom and autonomy of choice. Based on how one makes sense of the situation in which one finds oneself, they can chose to take a particular stance.

Freedom is at the core of human existence. It fosters an authentic stance towards values based on engagement and commitment. Man is what he does. The only reality is action. Man is nothing other than his own projects. Man exists only to the extent that he realises himself. Therefore, he is nothing more than the sum of his actions, nothing more than his life. We have choices to make, but life is an ever-evolving process. We also have the freedom to make further choices over time.

Conclusion

Working in the intensive care is exciting and often rewarding. However, it also repeatedly brings people face to face with existential issues. All of us are at the centre of our universe. Often it may feel like walking on a razor's edge or walking on a tight rope. Self-care and installing appropriate safety nets are important not only for our personal well-being but to be able to continue to play our chosen role effectively. Sometimes the margins between dis-ease and disease may be thin. When symptoms of dis-ease, often seen as burnout, worsen and become more persistent, it may be worth seeking help beyond mentorship, self-help and peer support.

References

1. Groopman JE. How doctors think. Mifflin: Houghton; 2007.
2. Kahneman D. Thinking, fast and slow. New York: Farrar, Straus and Giroux; 2011.
3. Kim K, Lee Y. Understanding uncertainty in medicine: concepts and implications in medical education. Korean J Med Educ. 2018;30(3):181–8. https://doi.org/10.3946/kjme.2018.92. PMID: 30180505. Published online

4. Cain S. Quiet: the power of introverts in a world that can't stop talking. London: Penguin Books; 2012.
5. Susman WI. Culture as history: the transformation of American society in the twentieth century. New York: Pantheon; 1984.
6. Allport GW. Personality: a psychological interpretation. New York: Holt; 1937.
7. Khanna R. Narratives of the mind: a new perspective on mental disorders. Sydney: Amazon Publishing; 2024.
8. Becker E. The birth and death of meaning: an interdisciplinary perspective on the problem of man. New York: The Free Press; 1962.
9. Lifton J. Death and identity. In: Fulton R, editor. Psychological effects of the atomic bomb in Hiroshima: the theme of death. New York: Wiley; 1976.
10. Orfi D. What doctors feel: how emotions affect the practice of medicine. Boston: Beacon Press; 2018.
11. Yalom ID. Love's executioner: and other tales of psychotherapy. New York: Basic Books; 1989.
12. Kishimi I, Koga F. The courage to be disliked: the Japanese phenomenon that shows you how to change your life and achieve real happiness. New York: Atria Books; 2018.
13. Kastenbaum RJ. Habituation as a model of human aging. Int J Aging Hum Dev. 1981;12(3):159–70.
14. Kihlstrom JF, Klein SB. Self-knowledge and self-awareness. Ann N Y Acad Sci. 1997;818(4):4–17.
15. Damasio A. Feelings of emotion and the self. Ann N Y Acad Sci. 2003;1001(1):253–61.

Chapter 18
Bouncing Safely Ahead: Contemplating the Future

Peter Vernon van Heerden (iD) and **Michael Ruppe** (iD)

> *Success is no accident. It is hard work, perseverance, learning, studying, sacrifice and, most of all, love of what you are doing or learning to do.*
>
> *– Pele*

Intensive care medicine is a relatively new specialty, with its inception borne from the need to support failing ventilation. The modern iteration truly took shape out of necessity with the advent of the polio epidemics of the 1950s. But it wasn't until the 1970s that it graduated to a more organized form as a stand-alone specialty [1]. We started as pioneers with a collective longing to give hope and healing to the sickest of the sick. With the subsequent 50 years of effort towards this shared goal, the intensivist of today finds themselves with a massive arsenal of technologies and resources at their disposal. The future is just as vibrant, with advances in pharmacology, machine learning and artificial intelligence being just a few of the possible sources of quantum leaps forward in the years to come.

Our workload has grown alongside our knowledge. Healthcare systems have expanded intensive care capacities, reshaping outpatient and daycare services and shifting traditional care to home settings (e.g. internal medicine, geriatrics, psychiatry). This expansion has dramatically reduced the instances where grief-stricken families are told, 'There is nothing more we can do'. Historically, this phrase offered intensivists an absolution that we are not afforded today. Intensivists can now place patients on life support in the form of extracorporeal membrane oxygenation (ECMO) when their hearts stop beating and have risen to unmeasurable heights of

P. V. van Heerden (✉)
Department of Anesthesiology, Critical Care and Pain Medicine,
Hadassah University Medical Center, Jerusalem, Israel

M. Ruppe
University of Louisville Department of Pediatrics, Division of Critical Care,
and Norton Children's Medical Group, Louisville, KY, USA
e-mail: michael.ruppe@louisville.edu

© The Author(s), under exclusive license to Springer Nature   193
Switzerland AG 2025
D. Dennis et al. (eds.), *Contemplating the Role of an Intensive Care Doctor*,
https://doi.org/10.1007/978-3-031-92766-9_18

coordinated critical care when faced with a global pandemic. Modern intensive care medicine always seems to find something more that can be done.

Today's intensivist practises in an era of previously unimaginable abilities. Lethal conditions in the past such as extreme prematurity, 'single ventricle' congenital heart disease, septic shock and multi-system organ failure, are no longer death sentences. It is the intensivist that conducts the orchestra of resuscitation, life support and often miraculous recovery. But woven into this reality is a spectre of mortality which remains a constant challenge.

The modern intensivist is also subject to ever-increasing oversight. Transparency in public reporting of clinical outcomes and national or global rankings of ICU performance are new realities to the intensivist. Reimbursement rates tied to performance metrics, benchmarking to compare outcomes between ICUs and 'scorecards' for doctors have added to the daily considerations that intensivists need to add to their careers [2–4]. This is what taxes us, as practitioners in the intensive care unit, as human beings.

Despite these challenges, over the past 50 years, we have also learnt that intensive care is a collective effort. Long gone are the days of the 'enthusiast' who chose to work in intensive care, as sometimes the sole provider, and who ruled with an iron fist, perhaps together with a small band of equally dedicated nursing staff. The history of intensive care is dominated by such giants of intensive care, who sacrificed much to advance the specialty. Today the therapeutic team in the intensive care unit includes doctors, nurses, allied health staff, respiratory therapists, social workers, nutritionists and more. In addition, consulting subspecialists play an integral role in the overall course of critically ill patients. Such a team still requires a leader, and it is the intensivist who shoulders both clinical responsibility and the well-being of the team.

Our profession is marked by remarkable capabilities and profound responsibilities. We shoulder an immense weight spread between making life-and-death decisions, serving as the leader of a collaborative team, tending to the psychosocial needs of the ICU and practising within the margins of a monitored healthcare system.

The above narrative puts into context the environment in which we go to work every day. As we confront challenges within a demanding yet fulfilling environment, it is crucial to acknowledge our humanity. When we interviewed intensivists, both in adult and pediatric practice, from Australia, the USA, and Israel a few years ago, we were struck by the commonality of challenges faced by intensive care doctors. Our findings from those interviews were published in several peer-reviewed papers and resulted in a book [5]. Those publications reported on our findings from the interviews but perhaps did not allow or encourage the reader to personally reflect on the findings.

This book is our attempt to use selected quotations from the initial interviews and build a framework for discussion and personal reflection. It has been divided into sections that explain the use of the book, raise the issues related to work as an intensivist, discuss the importance of communication and finally deal with how we should care for ourselves. The authors delve into the common human-factor issues we are faced with every day. The format of the book is such that each quotation and the questions raised can be used either for self-reflection or to stimulate a discussion with team members in the workplace.

We work hard in a demanding yet rewarding environment. We have the benefit of being an integral part of a therapeutic team, standing on the shoulders of giants who have taken intensive care medicine to unprecedented heights. This needs to be tempered by the fact that we are social human beings, privileged to be present at the crossroads of severe illness in patients in their most vulnerable moments. We are fiercely capable of practicing our trade but cannot deny that we are also emotional, feeling creatures with limits to our resilience. The format of the book encourages thinking about problems as an individual and discussing them with team members. We hope this book will help highlight some of the common issues we face in our work, allow us to delve a bit deeper into what each issue raises and perhaps gain a better understanding of ourselves and our field.

References

1. Grenvik A, Pinsky MR. Evolution of the intensive care unit as a clinical center and critical care medicine as a discipline. Crit Care Clin. 2009;25(1):239–50.
2. Lindenauer PK, Remus D, Roman S, Rothberg MB, Benjamin EM, Ma A. Bratzler DW *public reporting and pay for performance in hospital quality improvement*. N Engl J Med. 2007;356:486–96.
3. Fernando SM, Neilipovitz D, Sarti AJ, Rosenberg E, Ishaq R, Thornton M, Kim J. Monitoring intensive care unit performance—impact of a novel individualised performance scorecard in critical care medicine: a mixed-methods study protocol. BMJ Open. 2018;8:e019165.
4. Salluh JIF, Soares M, Keegan MT. Understanding intensive care unit benchmarking. Intensive Care Med. 2017;43:1703–7.
5. Dennis, D., Calhoun, A., Knott, C., Khanna, R., and van Heerden, P.V. "Stories from ICU doctors: navigating and conquering adversity" (2023).

Glossary[1]

Adverse event an unintended undesirable outcome of a medical intervention or decision

After-hours any time after routine daytime work hours

Anaesthesia the process of producing non-awareness to noxious stimuli, such as surgical incision

Anaesthesiologist the medical practitioner who administers medications to induce and maintain anaesthesia

Anaesthetist see Anaesthesiologist

Arrest cessation of function. May be cardiac due to absence of electrical activity (asystole) or chaotic electrical activity (e.g. ventricular fibrillation); or respiratory (breathing); or both

Attending in the context of this book, attending is sometimes used as a synonym for intensivist

BIPAP BiLevel positive airway pressure is a non-invasive ventilation therapy used to assist with breathing

Cachectic a condition characterized by weight loss, muscle wasting and loss of body fat

Cardiac arrest see **Arrest**

Cardiopulmonary arrest see **Arrest**

Cardiopulmonary resuscitation an emergency procedure that combines chest compressions with artificial breathing (ventilation) to manually preserve blood circulation and breathing in a person in cardiac arrest

Carcinoma cancer

---

[1]This glossary aims to provide consistency for terminology used in different geographical zones for the structure and practice of intensive care teams. The editors have purposefully standardized the terminology in the text to allow consistency around comparable roles or functions. It is not intended as advocacy to replace usual descriptive words in different geographical zones.

© The Editor(s) (if applicable) and The Author(s), under exclusive license to   197
Springer Nature Switzerland AG 2025
D. Dennis et al. (eds.), *Contemplating the Role of an Intensive Care Doctor*,
https://doi.org/10.1007/978-3-031-92766-9

Catheter a long hollow tube usually made of plastic/nylon which can be inserted into a body cavity

Central intravenous (IV) access see Central line; see IV

Central line a hollow plastic/nylon catheter placed into a large vein or the right atrium of the heart within the chest cavity via the internal jugular, subclavian, or femoral veins for the purpose of measuring venous pressures or administering medications.

Central line kit the equipment need to place a central ine in a safe and sterile manner

Cerebrospinal fluid (CSF) the clear, colourless fluid found within the brain and around the spinal cord, providing a barrier against mechanical shock

Clinician doctors and other medical and allied health personnel who are primarily occupied with patient care

Code another way of saying the patient has suffered a cardiac/cardiopulmonary arrest (he/she has 'coded')

Code cart resuscitation trolley containing all the equipment and medications required to manage acute resuscitation

College the body responsible for the training of intensive care specialists

College of Intensive Care of Australia and New Zealand see **College**

Compound fracture when there is an open wound or break in the skin near the fractured bone (broken bone)

Congenital heart disease where one or more problems with the heart's structure or function are present at birth

Consultant in the context of this book, consultant is sometimes used as a synonym for intensivist

CPR Acronym for 'cardiopulmonary resuscitation'

Critical care medicine the branch of medicine dealing primarily with organ support for patients with life-threatening conditions

CT scan Abbreviation of 'computed tomography' scan which refers to a computerized X-ray imaging procedure that rotates around the body to provide cross-sectional images or 'slice' images

Debrief; debriefing discussion after the event to clarify the issues surrounding the vent, such as causality and possible prevention in the future

Decompensation when there is a deterioration of a structure or system in the body that was previously working with the help of compensatory mechanisms such as medication

Disclosure revealing the details of an incident to all parties involved

Diuretic a medication used to increase fluid and salt output via the kidneys

Ebola a virus that causes a rare but severe illness in humans

ECMO extracorporeal membrane oxygenation, the removal of the blood from a patient, oxygenating it across a semi-permeable membrane and then returning the blood to the patient's circulation – a treatment which replaces the function of the lungs and/or heart artificially

Elective surgery surgery which is planned and is usually non-urgent (e.g. hernia repair)

Electrocardiogram (ECG or EKG) records the electrical signals in the heart to diagnose absent (asystole) or abnormal (dysrhythmia) heartbeats

Emergency medicine the branch of medicine which deals with all acute presentations to the hospital

Emergency Room (ER); Emergency Department (ED) the area of an acute hospital dealing with emergency care

Emotional Quotient (EQ) the level of a person's emotional intelligence

End-of-life care see **Palliative care**

Epi abbreviation of epinephrine, which is a hormone that normally regulates the sympathetic nervous system and prepares the body for action. During resuscitation it is commonly used to increase blood pressure, increase heart rate and improve cardiac output

Extracorporeal membrane oxygenation see **ECMO**

External ventricular drain (EVD) a flexible plastic catheter placed by a neurosurgeon to divert fluid from the ventricles of the brain and allow for monitoring of intracranial pressure. See **intracranial monitor**; see **intracranial pressure**

Faculty a sub-division of a college or university dealing with a defined subject, e.g. Faculty of Intensive Care Medicine

Fellow this has slightly different meanings in Australia/Britain where it refers to a trainee doctor who has completed training and examinations to be a specialist and, in the USA and Israel, where it means a doctor still in specialist training who is undertaking a period of study in a specific speciality

Frailty a decline in physical and cognitive reserves that leads to increased vulnerability

Glasgow Coma Scale (GCS) a scale use to measure the level of awareness of self and surroundings (may range from awake/conscious to drowsy to asleep to unconscious/comatose)

Goal(s) of Care the agreed and desirable outcomes of a specific treatment plan

Haemorrhagic shock; see also Uncompensated haemorrhagic shock a life-threatening medical condition where there is inadequate blood flow to the body's tissues due to excessive bleeding

Hospice an institution for providing palliative care for patients with terminal/end of life conditions

Human factors all the aspects of care that relate to human nature and human activity

ICU Acronym for 'intensive care unit'

Intelligence Quotient (IQ) a standardized measure of intelligence

Intensive Care Medicine see **critical care medicine**

Intensivist a medical doctor qualified in the independent practice of caring for critically unwell patients. Other terms used in the world are 'intensive care physician', 'intensive care attending', 'intensive care consultant'

Intercostal catheter also known as a chest tube, is a tube inserted into the chest to drain air or fluid from around the lungs

Intracranial bleed a brain bleed

Intracranial monitor a monitor that determines pressure of cerebrospinal fluid (CSF) within the brain

Intracranial pressure pressure of cerebrospinal fluid (CSF) within the brain

Intubated/intubation/intubating placing a hollow tube into the trachea/windpipe of a patient to facilitate connection to a mechanical ventilator

Invasive meaning entering a body space such as the chest or abdomen or a blood vessel

IV Abbreviation for administrating intravenous fluids or a 'drip' in lay terms

Lasix the trade name for furosemide/frusemide, a diuretic medication

M&M Acronym for '**Morbidity and Mortality' meetings** that discuss patient outcomes, particularly adverse events, complications and death

Mechanical ventilation the act of replacing or supporting the lung function of a patient using a machine (ventilator)

MICU Acronym for 'medical intensive care unit'

Morbidity and mortality meetings meetings held specifically to discuss adverse outcomes, either additional illness/burden or death

MRI Abbreviation for magnetic resonance imaging to produce high-quality radiological images

On-call being available in person or on the telephone to deal with urgent matters arising in the intensive care unit

Open disclosure see **Disclosure**

OR Acronym for 'operating room'

Oxygen monitoring measuring and displaying the results of the oxygen concentration or partial pressure in the blood either non-invasively (e.g. with a finger probe) or invasively (e.g. by taking repeated blood samples)

Oxygenation the state of the oxygen concentration or partial pressure in the blood of the patient

Palliative care providing care and symptom control for patients with terminal (end of life) conditions such as advanced malignancy

Pancreatectomy surgical removal of the pancreas, an organ of the digestive and endocrine systems

Pathogen any small viral or bacterial organism that can cause disease

Percutaneous via/through the skin of a patient

Peritoneal the space within the abdominal cavity

Physician a qualified medical doctor (in Britain/Australia it might also signify a specialist in internal medicine)

PICU Acronym for 'pediatric intensive care unit'

Post-traumatic stress disorder (PTSD) a psychological reaction to experiencing or witnessing a significantly traumatic or shocking event or series of events

Pneumothorax (singular); Pneumothoraces (pleural) collapsed lung or lungs

Proning where patients are positioned lying on their frontside (stomach-down) to facilitate the work of breathing. Proning was a commonly applied treatment during the COVID-19 pandemic to optimise oxygenation

Provider usually a registered medical professional entitled to provide medical services

PTSD see **Post-traumatic stress disorder**

Pulmonology the medical specialty dealing with lung diseases

Pupils fixed and dilated may be caused by various factors including head trauma, drug use and neurological conditions and may indicate a serious medical/neurological emergency

Recovery the area of the hospital where patients recover for a short period after a surgical procedure (recovery room) or the act of getting better from a certain condition or illness ('he recovered from pneumonia')

Registrar in Britain/Australia this means a junior/trainee doctor who is undertaking training in a medical specialty

Renal function the level of function of the kidneys

Resident in Israel/USA this has the same definition as **registrar** above, while in Britain/Australia it means a junior doctor before he/she enters specialist training (a rank below registrar)

Respiratory therapist an allied health professional who deals with treatments for the lung, such as oxygen therapy and mechanical ventilation

Resuscitation the act of providing urgent support for heart or lung function in the event of cardiac/cardiopulmonary arrest or urgent treatment of a life-threatening condition such as very low blood pressure due to sepsis

Root Cause Analysis careful analysis of an event or series of events in order to determine the underlying cause/s

Scan see **CT** and **MRI**

Scrubs the clothing often worn by physicians, nurses and other healthcare workers involved in patient care

Sedation protocol a systematic approach to safely administer medications to sedate patients during times of critical illness, surgery or painful procedures

Situational awareness knowing where you are and what is going on around you

Subarachnoid Haemorrhage a brain bleed that occurs between the brain and the tissues covering the brain

Suction applying negative pressure, e.g. via a tube to remove secretions from the patient's airway

Telemetry being able to view patient physiological parameters (e.g. blood pressure, heart rhythm) at a distance from the patient. This may be in another room or across the world

TGA abbreviation for Therapeutic Goods Administration which is the government agency enforcing the standards for therapeutic goods in Australia

Total Parental Nutrition (TPN) feeding that is provided intravenously, outside of the digestive tract

Trach short for tracheostomy

Tracheostomy the insertion of a hollow tube into the windpipe/trachea via an incision in the front of the neck

Trauma bay A treatment bay or bed area within an Emergency Department which is equipped to manage traumatic injuries

Trisomy 21 a genetic disorder also known as Down's syndrome, often involving defects in the heart

Uncompensated haemorrhagic shock a late phase of haemorrhagic shock where the body's compensatory mechanisms become inadequate. See **haemorrhagic shock**

Ventilator see **Mechanical ventilation**

Ward round a formalized bedside review of each patient in the ward by the medical team

Workup the procedures undertaken by doctors to arrive at a medical diagnosis, including history taking, laboratory tests, X-rays and other investigations

Index